刮痧图解
Illustrations of Guasha Therapy

主编 郑美凤 何芙蓉
主译 韩丑萍
英文主审 Lucy Dean

Chief Editors Zheng Mei-feng He Fu-rong
Chief Translator Han Chou-ping
Chief English Reviewer Lucy Dean

上海科学技术出版社
Shanghai Scientific and Technical Publishers

图书在版编目(CIP)数据

刮痧图解：汉英对照 / 郑美凤，何芙蓉主编；韩丑萍主译. —上海：上海科学技术出版社，2009.10
（汉英对照口袋书：彩图版）
ISBN 978-7-5323-9625-2

Ⅰ. 刮… Ⅱ. ①郑…②何…③韩… Ⅲ. 刮搓疗法－图解 Ⅳ. R244.4-64

中国版本图书馆 CIP 数据核字(2008)第 131851 号

上海世纪出版股份有限公司
上海 科 学 技 术 出 版 社   出版发行
（上海钦州南路71号 邮政编码200235）
新华书店上海发行所经销
浙江新华印刷技术有限公司印刷
开本 889×1194 1/64 印张 3.5
字数 158千字
2009年10月第1版   2011年1月第2次印刷
ISBN 978-7-5323-9625-2/R·2574
定价：30.00元

本书如有缺页、错装或坏损等严重质量问题，请向工厂联系调换

内容提要

刮痧疗法从中医学的整体观念出发,充分调动人体自身的积极因素,具有简便易行、安全可靠、效果显著、无不良反应等特点,是一种切实可行的绿色疗法。

本书共分上篇、下篇和附篇三个部分。上篇为刮痧基础理论,介绍刮痧疗法的基础理论,包括刮痧疗法简介、常用器具、基本步骤、常用的部位和穴位、操作方法及刮痧疗法的适应证和注意事项。下篇为刮痧疗法的实践应用,介绍常见临床病证的刮痧治疗和刮痧保健疗法。附篇为刮痧疗法验案介绍。

本书内容丰富,通俗易懂,可作为海内外广大临床医生、医学院校学生、留学生学习刮痧疗法的参考用书,亦可作为自我保健和治疗者的学习用书。

Synopsis of Contents

Based on the holistic view of traditional Chinese medicine, Guasha therapy can be used in a full range of treatments to promote the body's self-healing ability. It is regarded as a convenient and reliable therapy, since it is safe, effective, and easy to operate. In addition, it does not cause any adverse reactions or side effects.

This book consists of three parts. Part A contains the essential theory of Guasha, including a brief introduction, an overview of commonly used tools, basic procedures, body parts and points, operational methods, and indications as well as precautions. Part B contains the practical applications of Guasha therapy in the treatment of common conditions and in health care in general. Finally the attached chapter provides a collection of typical case studies illustrating the use of Guasha therapy.

With rich contents and straightforward descriptions, this book can serve as a sound reference book for clinicians, medical students and overseas students as well as those who are interested in self care and treatment.

目 录

上篇 刮痧疗法的基础理论

第一章 刮痧疗法简介 ——2
第二章 刮痧疗法常用的器具 ——8
第一节 刮痧用具 /8
第二节 刮痧介质 /10

第三章 刮痧疗法的步骤 ——12
第一节 持板法 /12
第二节 刮痧的范围 /13
第三节 常用刮痧法 /15
第四节 特殊刮痧法 /18

第四章 刮痧疗法常用的部位与穴位 ——20
第一节 背部与穴位 /20
第二节 头部与穴位 /27
第三节 颈部与穴位 /31
第四节 胸腹部与穴位 /32
第五节 四肢与穴位 /37
附：皮部分布图 /48

第五章 刮痧疗法实施前的准备 ——51
第一节 选穴原则 /51
第二节 配穴方法 /53

1

第三节 刮痧患者体位的选择 /55

第六章 刮痧疗法的操作方法 —— 59
　　第一节 施术前的操作 /59
　　第二节 施术中的操作 /60
　　第三节 施术后的操作 /62

第七章 刮痧疗法的适应证 —— 63

第八章 刮痧疗法的禁忌证与注意事项 —— 64

下篇 刮痧疗法的实践应用

第九章 内科病症的刮痧疗法应用 —— 68
　　第一节 中暑 /68
　　第二节 发热 /71
　　第三节 感冒 /74
　　第四节 咳嗽 /78
　　第五节 哮喘 /81
　　第六节 头痛 /86
　　第七节 失眠 /92
　　第八节 胁痛 /96
　　第九节 呕吐 /99
　　第十节 呃逆 /102
　　第十一节 胃痛 /106
　　第十二节 便秘 /110
　　第十三节 眩晕 /113
　　第十四节 高血压 /116
　　第十五节 面瘫 /120
　　第十六节 三叉神经痛 /123

第十章 骨伤外科病症的刮痧疗法应用 —— 127

第一节　落枕 /127

第二节　颈椎病 /130

第三节　扭伤、劳损 /134

第四节　肩凝证 /142

第五节　腰痛 /146

第六节　坐骨神经痛 /148

第七节　网球肘 /151

第八节　腓肠肌痉挛 /153

第十一章　妇儿科病症的刮痧疗法应用 —— 157

第一节　消化不良（食积）/157

第二节　百日咳 /160

第三节　痛经 /162

第四节　月经不调 /166

第五节　乳腺小叶增生 /169

第十二章　五官科病症的刮痧疗法应用 —— 172

第一节　目赤肿痛 /172

第二节　麦粒肿 /174

第三节　牙痛 /177

第四节　咽喉肿痛 /179

第十三章　刮痧疗法在美容保健方面的应用 —— 182

第一节　减肥 /182

第二节　脱发 /186

第三节　痤疮 /189

第四节　保健养生刮痧法 /191

附篇　刮痧疗法典型验案举隅

验案一　刮痧治疗失眠验案 /198

验案二　刮痧治疗胃痛验案 /200
验案三　刮痧治疗落枕验案 /201
验案四　刮痧治疗便秘验案 /203
验案五　刮痧治疗月经不调验案 /205
验案六　刮痧治疗小儿消化不良验案 /207

参考文献 —————————————————209

Contents

Part A　Essential Theory of Guasha Therapy

Chapter 1　Brief Introduction to Guasha Therapy ————— 4

Chapter 2　Common Tools of Guasha Therapy ————— 9

　Section 1　Guasha tools / 9

　Section 2　Guasha medium /11

Chapter 3　Procedures for Guasha Therapy ————— 13

　Section 1　Method for holding the Guasha board /13

　Section 2　Scope of Guasha /14

　Section 3　Common Guasha methods /17

　Section 4　Special Guasha methods /19

Chapter 4　Common Body Parts and Points Used in Guasha Therapy ————— 24

　Section 1　Back /24

　Section 2　Head /29

　Section 3　Neck /31

　Section 4　Chest and abdomen /36

Section 5　Four extremities /43

Attached: Profile of cutaneous regions /48

Chapter 5　Preparations Prior to Guasha Therapy —— 52

Section 1　Principle of point selection /52

Section 2　Method of point combination /54

Section 3　Selection of body position /58

Chapter 6　Operational Procedures of Guasha Therapy —— 60

Section 1　Procedures prior to Guasha therapy /60

Section 2　Procedures during Guasha therapy /61

Section 3　Procedures after Guasha therapy /62

Chapter 7　Indications for Guasha Therapy —— 63

Chapter 8　Precautions for Guasha Therapy —— 65

Part B　Guasha Therapy in Practice

Chapter 9　Guasha Therapy for Internal Diseases —— 70

Section 1　Sunstroke /70

Section 2　Fever /73

Section 3　Common cold /76

Section 4　Cough /80

Section 5　Asthma /85

Section 6　Headache /88

Section 7　Insomnia /95

Section 8　Hypochondriac pain /98

Section 9　Vomiting /101

Section 10　Hiccups /105

Section 11　Gastric pain /108

Section 12 Constipation /112

Section 13 Vertigo /114

Section 14 Hypertension /118

Section 15 Facial palsy /122

Section 16 Trigeminal neuralgia /125

Chapter 10 Guasha Therapy for Traumatology and External Conditions —— 129

Section 1 Stiff neck /129

Section 2 Cervical spondylosis /133

Section 3 Sprain or strain /141

Section 4 Frozen shoulder /144

Section 5 Lower back pain /147

Section 6 Sciatica /150

Section 7 Tennis elbow /152

Section 8 Sural spasm /155

Chapter 11 Guasha Therapy for Gynecological and Pediatric Conditions —— 159

Section 1 Dyspepsia (food retention) /159

Section 2 Whooping cough /161

Section 3 Dysmenorrhea /165

Section 4 Irregular menstruation /167

Section 5 Lobula hyperplasia of the mammary gland /170

Chapter 12 Guasha Therapy for Eye, Ear, Nose, and Throat Conditions —— 173

Section 1 Conjunctivitis /173

Section 2 Stye /175

Section 3　Toothache /178

Section 4　Sore throat /180

Chapter 13　Guasha Therapy for Cosmetology and Health Care —— 184

Section 1　Weight loss /184

Section 2　Hair loss /188

Section 3　Acne /190

Section 4　Guasha therapy for health preservation /194

Attached chapter　Case Studies of Guasha Therapy —— 197

Case report 1　Guasha therapy for insomnia /198

Case report 2　Guasha therapy for gastric pain /200

Case report 3　Guasha therapy for stiff neck /202

Case report 4　Guasha therapy for constipation /204

Case report 5　Guasha therapy for irregular menstruation /206

Case report 6　Guasha therapy for infantile dyspepsia /207

Reference —— 210

上篇 刮痧疗法的基础理论
Part A Essential Theory of Guasha Therapy

第一章 刮痧疗法简介

刮痧疗法，自古以来，流传民间，源远流长。多用于治疗夏秋季时病，如中暑、外感、胃肠道疾病等。远在盛唐时代，古籍就有以苎麻治疗痧病的记载。有人认为刮痧是由推拿手法衍变而来，《保赤推拿法》载："刮者，医指挨儿皮肤，略加力而下也。"元明时期，也有较多刮痧疗法的记载，称为"夏法"。嗣后，历代均有载录。清代郭志邃《痧胀玉衡》载："刮痧法，背脊颈骨上下，又胸前胁肋两背肩臂痧，用铜钱蘸香油刮之。"吴尚先《理瀹骈文》曰："阳痧腹痛，莫妙以瓷调羹蘸香油刮背，盖五脏之系，咸在于背；利之则邪气随降，病自松解。"千余年来，刮痧之法以其设备简单、操作简便、经济安全、适应证广、防治兼顾、疗效肯定、易学易懂，并具有祛邪外出、行气活血之奇功而传习效用。不仅成为民间疗法的精华，也成为中医学宝库中的一颗奇葩。近年来，刮痧疗法颇受广大医务工作者和民众的青睐，使这个流传久远的自然疗法与现代医学越来越重视的"回归自然"防治疾病思想相契合。

刮痧疗法属中医外治法的一种。在定义上有广义和狭义之分。主要用于治疗临床上称之为"痧症"的病证。广义的刮痧疗法包括刮痧、拧痧、挑痧、放血、放筋等；狭义刮痧疗法则仅指刮痧，即是指应用光滑的硬物器具或手指、金属针具等，在人体表面特定部位，反复进行刮、挤、揪、捏、刺等物理刺激，造成皮肤表面瘀血点、瘀血斑或点状出血，或配合应用一些中草药单方、验方，通过刺激皮部、体表络脉，通过经络的传导作用，激发人体内脏器官的协调功能，改善人体气血流通状态，从而达到平衡阴阳、扶正祛邪、排泄瘀毒、退热解惊、开窍益神等功效。

刮痧疗法的适应证，统称为痧证。中医学认为，痧证多由于风、湿、火三气相搏，当人体正气下降时，外袭肌肤，内郁阳气而为病。是夏秋季常见急性疾病，也可见于其他季节。临床以痧点（象），即施行刮痧疗法后，局部皮肤上很快出现的紫红色，类似细沙粒的累累出血点和局部或全身的酸胀感为主要表现。痧证可涉及临床内、外、妇、儿、五官等各科疾病，轻者影响身体健康、生活工作，重者出现胸闷烦躁、腹痛吐泻、口唇青紫，甚者昏厥而危及生命。有言"痧证多胀"，因而不同疾病引起的痧证中，多有头昏脑胀、胸部闷胀、腹部胀痛、全身酸胀等症状。有中暑引起的"暑痧"、"转筋痧"；呕吐腹泻，腓肠肌痉挛的"吊脚痧"；闭经吐血鼻衄、烦躁失眠等的"倒经痧"；小儿虫积、腹痛腹胀的"蛔结痧"；腰痛酸楚，小腿无力的"腰痛痧"，等等。

刮痧疗法是一种特殊的物理疗法。施术者借助工具，通过一定的手法，将力作用于患者身体的特定部位或穴位的肌肤，而达到治病强身的目的。现代医学研究认为，刮痧疗法可直接刺激皮肤的末梢神经，改善局部组织的血液、淋巴循环，增强新陈代谢，促进营养供给，并通过神经-内分泌-免疫调节网络，调节人体的免疫功能，增强机体的防御能力，达到改善病理状态，抑制病理过程的作用。是值得学习和推广的一种疗法。

Chapter 1 Brief Introduction to Guasha Therapy

With ancient origins and extensive development, Guasha therapy has been practiced consistently for thousands of years. 'Gua' means to scrape or rub, while 'Sha' is a reddish, elevated patch of skin. Sha is the term used to describe blood in the subcutaneous tissue that raises into a small red bump during Guasha therapy. It works well for seasonal diseases in summer or autumn such as sunstroke, external contraction, and gastrointestinal disorders. The records of using Guasha in the treatment of sunstroke with Ramee (zhù má, Boehmeria Nivea L. Gaud) can be traced back to the flourishing Tang dynasty. Some scholars believe that Guasha derives from tuina manipulations. The Tuina Manipulations for Raising and Protecting Children (bǎo chì tuī ná fǎ) by Xia Yun-ji in the Qing dynasty states that, 'Gua means applying a slightly heavier pressure with the physicians' fingers to the child's skin'. The records of the use of Guasha therapy are also available from the Yuan and Ming dynasties, referred to as summer therapy. After this time, the records of Guasha are preserved throughout the dynasties. For example, a systemic monograph on Guasha therapy called *the Guide to the Differential Diagnosis and Treatment of Exanthema and Filthy Diseases* (shā zhàng yù héng), by Guo Zhi-sui in the Qing dynasty, records that, 'Guasha therapy involves the layering of sesame oil on the skin and scraping the neck and back along the spine or chest area, bilateral hypochondriac area, shoulders, and arms with a copper coin'; and the *Rhymed Discourses*

Chapter 1 Brief Introduction to Guasha Therapy

on External Therapy (lǐ yuè pián wén), by Wu Shang-xian in the Qing dynasty, records that, 'For abdominal pain due to yang Sha, a miraculous treatment method is to scrape the back with a porcelain spoon dipped in sesame oil, since the back-Shu points connect with all the five-zang organs. Scraping these points can remove pathogenic qi and thus benefit the patient'. The advantages of Guasha include simple tools, easy operation, low cost, extensive indications and efficacy for prevention and treatment. For these reasons, Guasha therapy has been practiced for thousands of years as a key part of TCM and other therapies. It has become especially popular among medical workers and the general public in recent years, partly as this age enduring natural therapy adheres to the call for biomedicine to return to nature.

Guasha is one of the external therapies of traditional Chinese medicine. Its definition is both broad and far reaching, and detailed. It is mainly indicated for disorders of 'Sha symptoms'. The broader use of Guasha includes scraping, twisting, pricking, blood-letting, and tendon relaxation, however, it is often used to refer to scraping alone: exertion of physical stimulations to specific body parts by scraping, squeezing, grasping, pinching and pricking with smooth, hard tools, fingers or metal needles. This causes spots, patches or punctuate bleeding on the body surface. Guasha therapy may be combined with a single recipe or common herbal formula to stimulate the cutaneous region and collaterals in order to activate internal organs through the meridian system. The result of Guasha therapy is to improve qi flow and blood circulation, balance yin and yang, strengthen the anti-pathogenic qi, remove pathogenic factors, discharge or drain stagnant toxins, clear heat, open the orifices, and refresh the mind.

The indications of Guasha therapy are generalized as Sha

syndrome. TCM asserts that Sha syndrome occurs as a result of internal obstruction of yang-qi from a decrease in the body's anti-pathogenic qi, coupled with external contraction of wind, dampness, and fire. It mainly manifests as acute conditions in summer and autumn, but may be present in other seasons. Sha syndrome is clinically characterized by Sha spots (exanthema), occurring immediately after treatment, purple, red and sand granule-sized petechia, or soreness and distension either local or generalized. It may involve a variety of clinical subspecialties such as internal medicine, external medicine, gynecology, pediatrics and ophthalmology & otorhinolaryngology. Mild conditions may affect the patients' health, life, and work, whereas a severe condition may cause chest tightness, vexations, abdominal pain, vomiting, diarrhea, cyanosis of lips, or even life-threatening fainting. There is Chinese saying that 'distension always accompanies Sha syndrome'. This is seen in clinic as patients with Sha syndrome always present with symptoms such as dizziness, head distension, chest oppression and distension, abdominal distension and pain, and general soreness or distension. Examples of this include 'summer-heat Sha' or 'muscle spasm Sha' due to sunstroke; 'cramp in cholera morbus' involving calf cramp due to vomiting and diarrhea; 'inverted menstruation' involving hematemesis, nosebleed, restlessness, and insomnia due to amenorrhea; infantile 'eruptive ascarides' characterized by intestinal parasitosis and abdominal pain or distension; and 'eruptive lumbago' characterized by lumbar soreness, pain, and weakness of the lower legs.

Guasha therapy is a special physical therapy. The Guasha practitioner exerts force on specific body parts or points with tools or hand manipulation to treat disorders and strengthen the body.

Biomedical studies show that Guasha therapy can directly stimulate subcutaneous peripheral nerves, improve local circulation of blood and lymph fluid, speed up the metabolism, promote nutritional supply, regulate immune function through the nerve-endocrine-immunoregulation network and facilitate the body's defensive abilities. This, thereby, improves the pathological state and suppresses the pathological process. Guasha, therefore, constitutes an important part of the study and application of Chinese medicine.

第二章 | 刮痧疗法常用的器具

第一节 刮痧用具

1. 刮痧板：是目前最常用的刮痧用具，多为水牛角等动物角质类制品，具有一定的硬度、弹性和韧性。也有以陶瓷、玉石等做成刮痧板，但都因易碎又容易刮伤皮肤或价格昂贵而难以普及。刮痧板的形状大同小异。多呈长方形，也有呈不规则形状，但多一侧棱角较薄，一侧棱角较厚。（图1～4）

2. 苎麻：是较早使用的工具。选取已经成熟的苎麻，去皮、枝叶并晒干，用根部较粗的纤维，捏成一团，在冷水里蘸湿即可使用。

3. 头发：取长头发，揉成一团，蘸香油，作工具使用。

此外，还有以陶瓷类（汤匙或瓶块）、木质类（如木梳）、贝壳类（蛤壳）、钱币类（铜钱、硬币）制成的刮痧用具等。（图5～8）

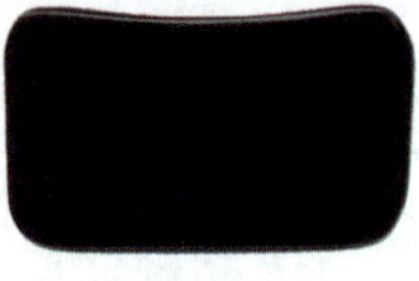

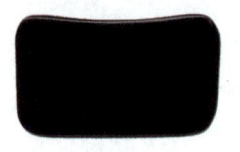

图1 长方形刮痧板
Fig.1 Rectangle board

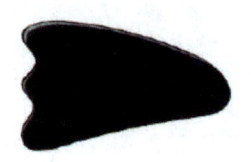

图2 不规则形刮痧板
Fig.2 Irregular-shaped board

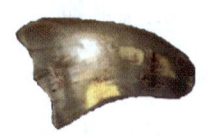

图3 水牛角刮痧板
Fig.3 Buffalo horn board

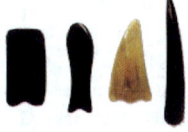

图4 不同形状刮痧板
Fig. 4 Different shapes of board

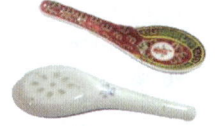

图5 汤匙
Fig.5 Soup spoon

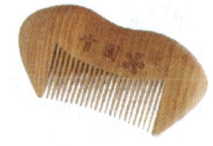

图6 木梳
Fig.6 Wooden comb

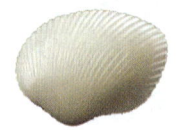

图7 贝壳
Fig.7 Shell

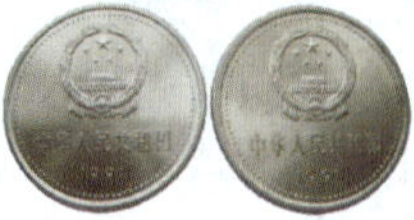

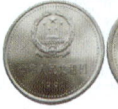

图8 硬币
Fig.8 Coin

Chapter 2 Common Tools of Guasha Therapy

Section 1 Guasha tools

1. Guasha boards: Guasha boards are the most commonly used tools. The boards are usually made of animal horn products such as buffalo. These boards are hard, elastic and flexible. Porcelain and jade boards are sometimes used for Guasha, however, these materials are

not popular since they are brittle, expensive, and may easily cause injury to the skin. The Guasha boards may be rectangle or irregular. Most boards have a thinner edge on one side and a thicker one on the other side. (See examples in Fig.1-4)

2. Ramee: This was a Guasha tool used in earlier times. Method: Select and decorticate the ripe ramee; remove the branches and leaves and dry in the sun; and then twist the fibers with thick roots and dip into the cold water.

3. Hair: Twist long hair and dip it into the sesame oil.

In addition, the following things can also be used as Guasha tools: porcelain (soup spoon or rice pot), wood (wooden comb), shell (clam shell), and coin (copper coin). (See examples in Fig.5-8)

第二节　刮痧介质

刮痧过程中，常在刮具和患者的刮拭部位涂抹一些具有润滑作用的物质，以利于手法的施行。常用的刮痧介质有以下几类，可根据具体病症灵活选用。

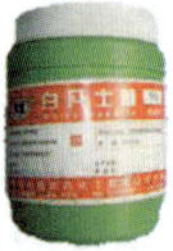

图9 凡士林
Fig. 9 Vaseline

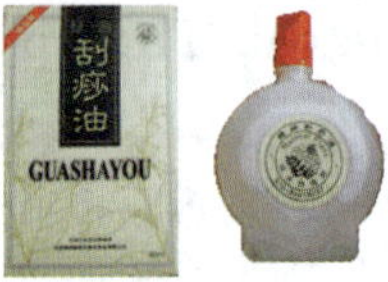

图10 刮痧油(1)
Fig.10 Guasha oil (1)

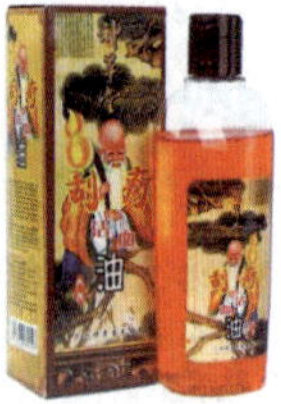

图11 刮痧油(2)
Fig.11 Guasha oil (2)

1.液体类：目前常用的刮痧液体介质如水、麻油、白酒、红花油、紫草油、万花油及一些特制的刮痧油等。

2.固体类：如冬青膏、凡士林、霜类等。

3.药剂类：如止痛灵、葱姜汁、薄荷水，根据临床症候辨证而特制的活血化瘀中草药制剂等。

其中以刮痧油最为常用。（图9～11）

Section 2 Guasha medium

Lubricating media are always applied to the Guasha tools and patients' skin for smooth manipulation. A variety of substances can be used on the basis of specific problems. The most common substances are as follows:

1. Liquid: The common liquid media include water, sesame oil, distillate spirit, safflower oil, pearl plant oil, and specially-made Guasha oil.

2. Solid: The common solid media includes holly ointment, Vaseline, and creams.

3. Drug agents: The common medical agents include Ethbenzamide, green onion and ginger juice, mint water, and Chinese medicinal preparations that act to activate blood and resolve stasis.

The Guasha oil is the most common medium. (See examples in Fig.9-11)

第三章 刮痧疗法的步骤

第一节 持板法

施术者肩、肘、腕自然弯曲,握空拳,刮板置于拇指和其他四指之间。刮板与选刮部位的皮肤吸附、紧贴并与刮拭方向保持45°~90°。刮拭时用力均匀,长度适中。以治疗为目的时,以刮板薄的一侧对着患者的皮肤;保健时,则以刮板厚的一侧紧贴被刮的部位。(图12~15)

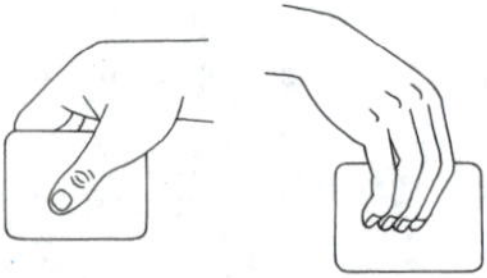

图12 持板法
Fig.12 Method for holding the board

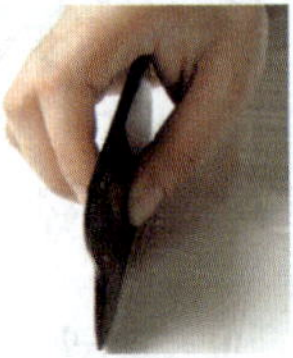

图13 持板侧面观
Fig.13 Side view

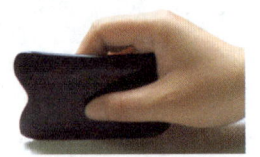

图14 持板前面观
Fig.14 Front view

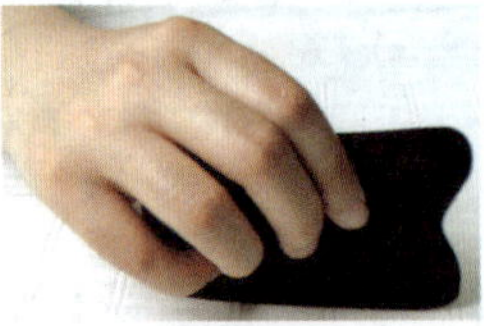

图15 持板背面观
Fig.15 Back view

Chapter 3　Procedures for Guasha Therapy

Section 1 Method for holding the Guasha board

The practitioner should naturally flex the shoulder, elbow, and wrist; make a hollow fist and put the board between thumb and the other four fingers; apply the board to the selected area and maintain an angle of 45°−90° towards the scraping direction; exert even and moderate-length force. For treatment of pathology, the thinner edge of the board is used to contact the skin; and for health preservation, the thicker edge of the board is used. (See examples in Fig.12-15)

第二节　刮痧的范围

刮痧的范围一般都以"点"、"线"结合以达到"面"的效果，并根据临床病情的变化而定。通常以尽量拉长其刮拭的范围为佳，临床上常见以下几种：

1. 线状：直线刮拭，即从一点向远处呈直线刮拭，临床常用于刮拭前、后头部、前额、面部、颈项部、胸背部、上下肢等部位；弧线刮拭，即从一点向远处呈抛物线样刮拭。多用于颞部、颈项至上背部、下颌及关节部位。（图16）

2. 放射状：扇形放射状刮拭，即刮拭时从一点向多方向呈扇形放射，多用于侧头部、后枕部；星状放射（环状）刮拭，即从一个局部向周围呈环状刮拭，多用于头的巅顶部或痛点比较固定

的部位。(图17)

3. 点状：刮拭局限于局部。多见病位明确或痛点明显的部位以及穴位的刮拭。(图18)

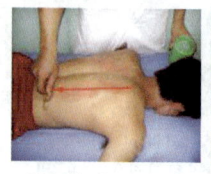

图16 直线刮拭
Fig.16 Straight line scraping

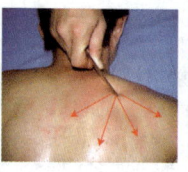

图17 放射状刮拭
Fig.17 Radiated scraping

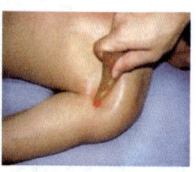

图18 点状刮拭
Fig.18 Punctiform scraping

Section 2 Scope of Guasha

Based on the presenting clinical condition, the application of Guasha generally works on 'spots' and 'lines', eventually resulting in a 'planar' effect. Better effect can be obtained by extending the application of Guasha. The common methods of application are as follows:

1. Linear: To scrape from a specific spot to other areas in a straight line, for example, on the anterior and posterior parts of the head, forehead, face, neck and nape, chest and back, and upper and lower extremities. Alternatively, one can scrape from a specific spot to other areas in a parabola, for example, on the temporal region, on the nape towards the upper back, lower mandible, and joints. (See Fig.16)

2. Radiated: To scrape from a specific spot in multiple directions creating a fan-shaped area, for example, on the lateral head or occipit. Alternatively, one can scrape from a specific spot to peripheral area in a circular manner, for example, on the vertex or on an area of fixed

pain. (See Fig. 17)

3. Punctiform: To scrape the local area, for example, in specific disease location or obvious tenderness spots as well as acupuncture points. (See Fig. 18)

第三节　常用刮痧法

1. 循经刮痧法

（1）刮板与刮拭方向呈30°~60°，均匀用力刮拭。用于身体较为平坦的部位经络刮拭。（图19）

（2）刮板与刮拭方向呈90°，刮板垂直、紧贴皮肤，并以一定压力快速、短距离的循经刮拭。（图20）

（3）按经络的走向循经长距离刮拭，用力轻柔、速度和缓、连绵不断，多用于刮拭结束时或用于调整经络、放松肌肉、消除疲劳等保健刮痧。（图21）

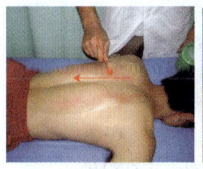

图19 30°~60°循经刮拭　　图20 90°循经刮拭　　图21 循经长距离刮拭
Fig.19 30°- 60° meridian scraping　Fig.20 90° meridian scraping　Fig.21 Extended meridian scraping

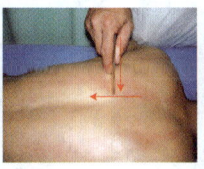

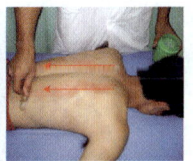

2. 穴位刮痧法

（1）刮板与刮拭方向保持45°。多用于骨骼、关节等角度部位穴位的刮拭。（图22）

（2）刮板与刮拭部位低于30°，吸定于皮肤上，用力由轻至重，做柔和而慢速的旋转按揉。多用于特定的穴位或痛点。（图23）

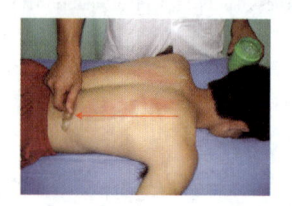

图22 45°穴位刮拭
Fig.22 45° scraping

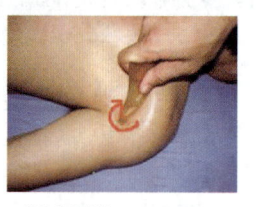

图23 旋转按揉
Fig.23 Rotated pressing and kneading

3. 局部刮痧法

（1）刮板与刮拭部位呈90°进行刮拭。操作时刮板垂直向下，逐渐用力，由轻至重，最后暂停片刻后突然抬起，可根据病情重复多次。多用于刮拭肌肉肥厚部位或穴位凹陷处。（图24）

（2）以刮板平面拍打而下以刺激部位，也可用五指或手掌自然弯曲拍打。多用于肘窝或腘窝处。（图25）

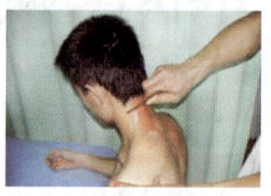

图24 90°刮拭
Fig.24 90° scraping

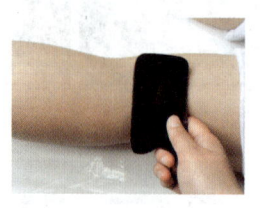

图25 拍痧
Fig.25 Tapping

Section 3 Common Guasha methods

1. Scraping along the meridians

1.1 Apply even force at an angle of 30°－60° between the Guasha board and the forward direction. This method is used for flat areas of the body. (See Fig.19)

1.2 Hold the board perpendicular to the skin, use a degree of pressure and scrape a short distance rapidly along the meridians, maintaining an angle of 90° throughout. (See Fig. 20)

1.3 Scrape a long distance along the pathway of the meridians with moderate-speed, a gentle and continuous force. This method is usually used at the end of the Guasha treatment or for preservation of health by regulating the meridians, relaxing muscles and relieving fatigue. (See Fig. 21)

2. Scraping the acupuncture points

2.1 Scrape points located at the axial areas or joints at an angle of 45° between the Guasha board and forward direction. (See Fig.22)

2.2 Maintain an angle of less than 30° between the Guasha board and the skin, apply the board to the skin, using gradually increasing force and combine with soft, slow, rotating pressure and kneading. This method is usually used for specific points or tender spots. (See Fig.23)

3. Scraping the local area

3.1 Scrape at an angle of 90° between the Guasha board and the skin using gradually increasing force, pause for a moment and then suddenly lift the board off the skin. This method is usually used for fleshy points or areas and can be repeated several times. (See Fig. 24)

3.2 Certain areas can be stimulated by tapping with the board, five fingers or a naturally flexed palm. This method is usually used in the cubital or popliteal fossa. (See Fig.25)

第四节 特殊刮痧法

特殊刮痧法流行于民间。如拧痧法（图26）：即与刮痧法相类似，但操作更为简便。施术者以示、中指相并屈曲，蘸清水，后拧夹穴位的皮肤，拧起后让手指滑下，如此反复，一般每次拧20下左右，以皮肤出现红色或紫色痧痕为度。若施术者手指水干后，可反复蘸湿，以减轻患者的疼痛。此法多用于对于痧证有特效的穴位，如印堂、风府、大椎、风池、曲泽、委中、缺盆等。

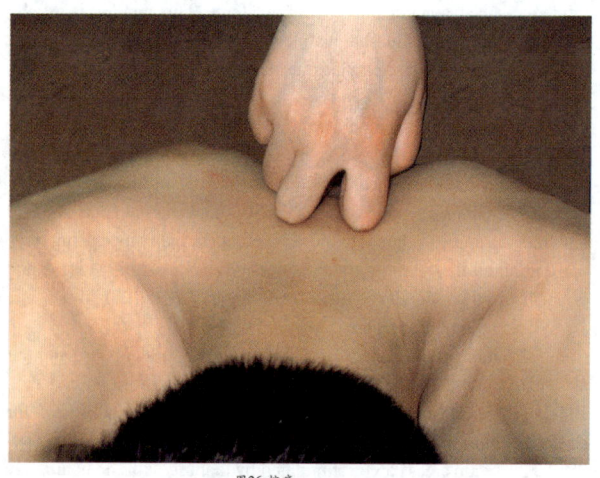

图26 拧痧
Fig.26 Twisting method

Section 4 Special Guasha methods

Some special Guasha methods are practiced in folk communities, for instance, twisting method (See Fig. 26). This is similar to Guasha but is more easily operated. Procedure: Flex the index and middle fingers; dip the proximal phalange into water; and pinch or twist the skin over the intended point and then loosen the fingers after twisting. This method can be done about 20 times each time until the local skin turns red or purple spots appear. The practitioner should keep the fingers wet to reduce pain. This method is usually used for special points such as Yintang (EX HN 3), Fengfu (GV 16), Dazhui (GV 14), Fengchi (GB 20), Quze (PC 3), Weizhong (BL 40) and Quepen (ST 12).

第四章　刮痧疗法常用的部位与穴位

第一节　背部与穴位

患者可取侧卧或俯卧位，也可伏坐于椅背上。先从第七颈椎起，沿督脉由上而下至第五腰椎；然后再从脊椎与肩胛内侧之间的区域，脊椎两侧由上而下至腰间；最后第一胸椎至第五腰椎旁开沿肋间向外侧斜刮。此即是最主要和常用的刮痧部位。（图27~29）

1. 天柱：后发际正中旁开1.3寸。
2. 大椎：背后，第七颈椎棘突下凹陷中。
3. 颈部夹脊穴区：颈部各脊椎棘突下两侧旁开0.5寸。
4. 肩井：大椎与肩峰之间。
5. 天宗：肩胛冈下窝中点。
6. 秉风：肩胛冈上窝中央，天宗穴直上。
7. 大杼：第一胸椎棘突下旁开1.5寸。
8. 风门：上背部，第二胸椎棘突下旁开1.5寸。
9. 肺俞：第三胸椎棘突下，旁开1.5寸。
10. 心俞：第五胸椎棘突下旁开1.5寸。
11. 至阳：背部，第七胸椎棘突下凹陷处。
12. 膈俞：第七胸椎棘突下旁开1.5寸。
13. 肝俞：第九胸椎棘突下旁开1.5寸。

第四章　刮痧疗法常用的部位与穴位
Chapter 4 Common Body Parts and Points Used in Guasha Therapy

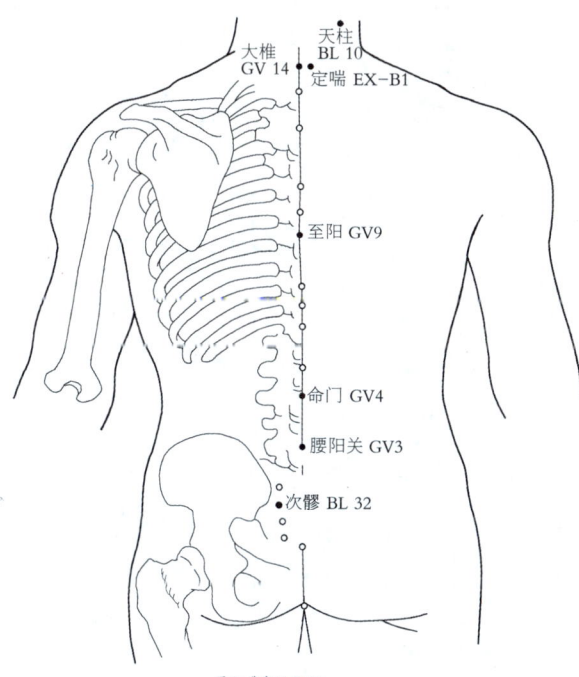

图27 背部穴位(1)
Fig.27 Points on the back (1)

14. 脾俞：第十一胸椎棘突下旁开1.5寸。
15. 胃俞：第十二胸椎棘突下旁开1.5寸。
16. 膏肓俞：第四胸椎棘突下旁开3寸。
17. 三焦俞：第一腰椎棘突下旁开1.5寸。

- 大杼 BL 11
- 风门 BL 12
- 肺俞 BL 13
- 心俞 BL 15
- 膈俞 BL 17
- 肝俞 BL 18
- 胆俞 BL 19
- 脾俞 BL 20
- 胃俞 BL 21
- 肾俞 BL 23
- 大肠俞 BL 25

图28 背部穴位(2)
Fig.28 Points on the back (2)

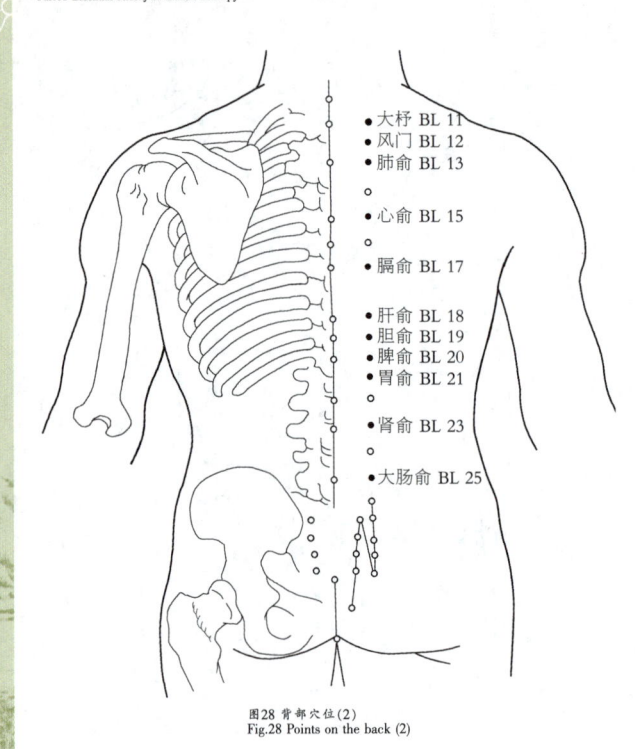

18. 肓门：腰部，第一腰椎棘突下旁开3寸。
19. 肾俞：第二腰椎棘突下旁开1.5寸。
20. 命门：第二腰椎棘突下。

第四章 刮痧疗法常用的部位与穴位
Chapter 4 Common Body Parts and Points Used in Guasha Therapy

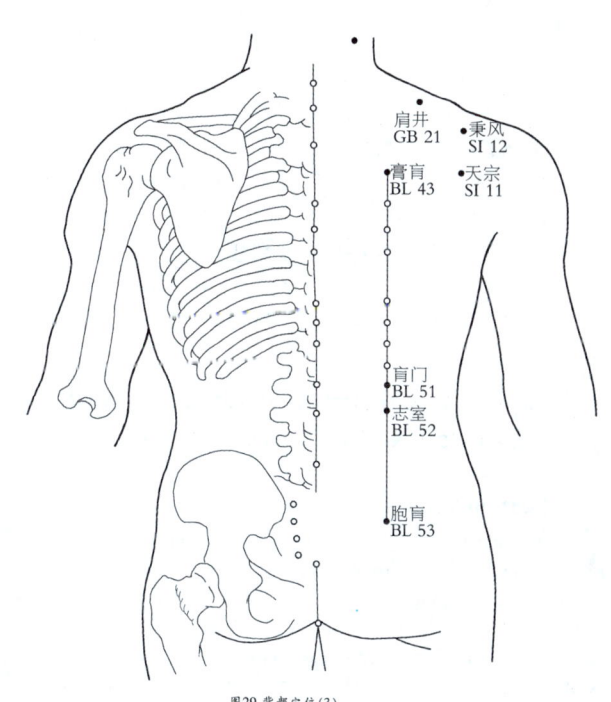

肩井 GB 21
秉风 SI 12
膏肓 BL 43
天宗 SI 11
肓门 BL 51
志室 BL 52
胞肓 BL 53

图29 背部穴位(3)
Fig.29 Points on the back (3)

21. 志室：第二腰椎棘突下旁开3寸。
22. 大肠俞：第四腰椎棘突下，旁开1.5寸。
23. 胞肓：臀部，平第二骶后孔，骶正中嵴旁开3寸。

24. 背俞穴：脊椎各棘突下两侧旁开1.5寸，与正中线平行的直线上。

25. 夹脊穴：背部正中，各椎体棘突下两侧旁开0.5寸。

26. 次髎：骶部，第二骶后孔中，髂后上棘内下方。

27. 八髎穴区：骶部，髂后上棘与正中线之间，平第一、第二、第三、第四骶后孔。

28. 腰阳关：第四腰椎棘突下凹陷处。

29. 腰眼：第四腰椎棘突下，旁开约3.5寸凹陷处。

30. 秩边：平第四骶后孔，骶正中嵴旁开3寸。

Chapter 4 Common Body Parts and Points Used in Guasha Therapy

Section 1 Back

The patient can adopt a lying position, either on the side or prone, or a head-down sitting position. The practitioner can scrape from C_7 to L_5 along the spine; then scrape the area between the spine and medical aspect of the scapula, or from bilateral sides of the spine to lumbar area; and finally scrape obliquely from the lateral borders of the vertebra T_1-T_5 toward the axillary line, along the intercostal spaces. These areas are the main and most commonly used areas for Guasha therapy. (See Fig.27-29)

1. Tianzhu (BL 10): Located 1.3 cun lateral to the midline of the posterior hairline.

2. Dazhui (GV 14): Located in the depression below the spinous process of C_7.

3. Cervical Jiaji (EX-B 2) points: Located 0.5 cun lateral to the spinous process of each vertebra.

4. Jianjing(GB 21): Located in between Dazhui(GV 14) and acromion.

5. Tianzong (SI 11): Located at the center of infrascapular fossa.

6. Bingfeng (SI 12): Located at the center of suprascapular fossa, directly above Tianzong (SI 11).

7. Dazhu (BL 11): Located 1.5 cun lateral to the spinous process of T_1.

8. Fengmen (BL 12): Located 1.5 cun lateral to the spinous process of T_2.

9. Feishu (BL 13): Located 1.5 cun lateral to the spinous process of T_3.

10. Xinshu (BL 15): Located 1.5 cun lateral to the spinous process of T_5.

11. Zhiyang (GV 9): Located in the depression below the spinous process of T_7.

12. Geshu (BL 17): Located 1.5 cun lateral to the spinous process of T_7.

13. Ganshu (BL 18): Located 1.5 cun lateral to the spinous process of T_9.

14. Pishu (BL 20): Located at 1.5 cun lateral to the spinous process of T_{11}.

15. Weishu (BL 21): Located 1.5 cun lateral to the spinous process of T_{12}.

16. Gaohuangshu (BL 43): Located 3 cun lateral to the spinous process of T_4.

17. Sanjiaoshu (BL 22): Located 1.5 cun lateral to the spinous process of L_1.

18. Huangmen (BL 51): Located 3 cun lateral to the spinous process of L_1.

19. Shenshu (BL 23): Located 1.5 cun lateral to the spinous process of L_2.

20. Mingmen (GV 4): Located in the depression below the spinous process of L_2.

21. Zhishi (BL 52): Located 3 cun lateral to the spinous process of L_2.

22. Dachangshu (BL 25): Located 1.5 cun lateral to the spinous process of L_4.

23. Baohuang (BL 53): Located 3 cun lateral to the median sacral crest, at the level of the second posterior sacral foramen.

24. Back-Shu points: Located 1.5 cun lateral to the spinous process of each vertebra, in a line paralleled to the midline.

25. Huatuo Jiaji (EX-B 2) points: Located 0.5 cun lateral to the spinous process of each vertebra.

26. Ciliao (BL 32): Located in the second sacral foramen, and at the medial and inferior aspect of the posterior superior iliac spine.

27. Baliao area: Located at the level of the first, second, third, and fourth sacral foramen, and in between the posterior superior iliac spine and the midline, altogether 8 points bilaterally.

28. Yaoyangguan (GB 3): Located in the depression below the spinous process of T_4.

29. Yaoyan (EX-B 7): Located approximately 3.5 cun lateral to the spinous process of T_4.

30. Zhibian (BL 54): Located 3 cun lateral to the median sacral crest.

第二节　头部与穴位

（图30～32）

1. 水沟：人中沟上1/3与下2/3交点。
2. 印堂：两眉连线的中点。
3. 太阳：眉梢与目外眦连线中点向后1寸。
4. 百会：两耳尖直上，前后正中线交点。
5. 四神聪：头顶，百会前后左右各旁开1寸。（图137）
6. 神庭：前发迹正中上0.5寸。
7. 率谷：两耳尖直上入发迹1.5寸。
8. 头临泣：头部，瞳孔直上入发迹0.5寸。
9. 头维：头侧部，额角发迹上0.5寸。
10. 上星：前额部，正中入发迹1寸。
11. 翳风：耳垂后方，平耳垂。
12. 颊车：面颊部，咀嚼时咬肌隆起，按之凹陷处。
13. 颧髎：面部，目外眦直下，颧骨下缘凹陷处。
14. 四白：瞳孔直下，眶下缘之间。
15. 阳白：瞳孔直上，眉上1寸。
16. 迎香：鼻翼旁开0.5寸。
17. 承浆：下颏，颏唇沟中点。
18. 地仓：口角外侧，瞳孔直下。
19. 攒竹：眉头凹陷。
20. 丝竹空：眉梢凹陷。
21. 鼻通：鼻甲软骨与鼻甲的交界处，近鼻唇沟上端处。

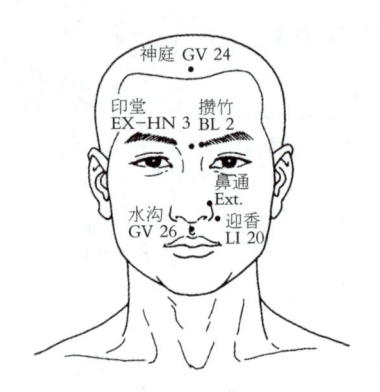

上篇 刮痧疗法的基础理论
Part A Essential Theory of Guasha Therapy

图30 头面颈项部穴位(1)
Fig.30 Points on the head, face and neck (1)

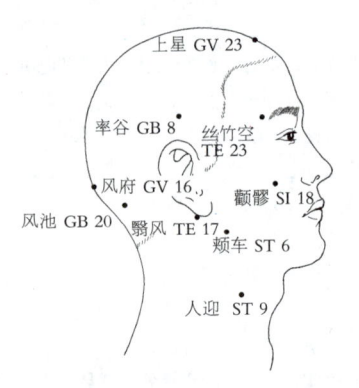

神庭 GV 24
印堂 EX-HN 3
攒竹 BL 2
鼻通 Ext.
水沟 GV 26
迎香 LI 20

图31 头面颈项部穴位(2)
Fig.31 Points on the head, face and neck (2)

上星 GV 23
率谷 GB 8
丝竹空 TE 23
风府 GV 16
颧髎 SI 18
风池 GB 20
翳风 TE 17
颊车 ST 6
人迎 ST 9

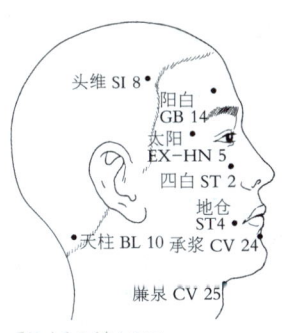

图32 头面颈项部穴位(3)
Fig.32 Points on the head, face, and neck (3)

Section 2 Head

(See Fig. 30-32)

1. Renzhong (GV 26): Located at the crossing point of the upper 1/3 and lower 2/3 of the philtrum.

2. Yintang (EX-HN 3): Located midway between the medial ends of the two eyebrows.

3. Taiyang (EX-HN 5): Located in the depression on the temple, approximately 1 cun posterior to the midpoint of the line connecting the end of eyebrow and the outer canthus.

4. Baihui (GV 20): Located at the midpoint of the line connecting the apexes of the two auricles.

5. Sishencong (EX-HN 1): A group of 4 points, at the vertex, 1 cun respectively posterior, anterior, and lateral to Baihui (GV 20). (See Fig. 137)

6. Shenting (GV 24): Located 0.5 cun directly above the midpoint of the anterior hairline.

7. Shuaigu (GB 8): Located 1.5 cun within the hairline, directly above the apex of the auricle.

8. Toulinqi (GB 15): Located 0.5 cun within the hairline, directly above the pupil.

9. Touwei (ST 8): Located 0.5 cun within the hairline and 4.5 cun lateral to Shenting (GV 24).

10. Shangxing (GV 23): Located 1 cun directly above the midpoint of the anterior hairline.

11. Yifeng (SJ 17): Located in the depression between the mandible and mastoid process, on a level with the ear lobe.

12. Jiache (ST 6): Located 1 finger-breadth anterior and superior to the lower angle of the mandible, at the prominence of the masseter muscle attachment when the teeth are clenched.

13. Quanliao (SI 18): Located directly below the outer canthus, in the depression on the lower border of zygoma.

14. Sibai (ST 2): Located directly below the center of the, in the depression at the infraorbital foramen.

15. Yangbai (GB 14): Located 1 cun directly above the midpoint of the eyebrow.

16. Yingxiang (LI 20): Located 0.5 cun lateral to ala nasi.

17. Chengjiang (CV 24): Located in the center of the mentolabial groove.

18. Dicang (ST 4): Located lateral to the corner of the mouth, directly below the pupil.

19. Cuanzhu (BL 2): Located on the medial extremity of the eyebrow.

20. Sizhukong (SJ 23): Located in the depression at the lateral end of the eyebrow.

21. Bitong (Extra): Located at the junction of the nasal bone

cartilage and nasal bone, near the superior extremity of the nasolabial groove.

第三节 颈部与穴位

（图31，27，32，34）

1. 风池：项后枕骨下两侧凹陷处。
2. 风府：项后，枕外粗隆上缘凹陷。
3. 定喘：大椎旁开0.5寸。
4. 廉泉：颈部，结喉上方，舌骨上缘凹陷处。
5. 缺盆：锁骨上窝的中点。
6. 人迎：颈部两侧，双肩膀筋部（胸锁乳突肌），或喉头两侧。

Section 3 Neck

(See Fig. 31, 27, 32, 34)

1. Fengchi (GB 20): Located in the depression between the upper portion of sternocleidomastoid and trapezius muscles, at the same level as Fengfu (GV 16).

2. Fengfu (GV 16): Located in the depression of the lower border of external occipital protuberance.

3. Dingchuan (EX-B 1): Located at 0.5 cun lateral to Dazhui (GV 14).

4. Lianquan (CV 23): Located above the Adam's apple, in the depression superior to the upper border of the hyoid bone.

5. Quepen (ST 12): Located at the midpoint of the supraclavicular fossa.

6. Renying (ST 9): Located level with the tip of the Adam's apple, on the anterior border of sternocleidomastoid muscle.

第四节 胸腹部与穴位

(图33~35)

1. 天突：胸骨上窝凹陷处。
2. 膻中：前正中线，平第四肋间。
3. 璇玑：胸部天突下1寸。
4. 中府：前正中线旁开6寸，平第一肋间隙。
5. 期门：乳头直下，第六肋间隙。
6. 梁门：脐上4寸，旁开2寸。
7. 腹通谷：脐上5寸，旁开0.5寸。
8. 大横：脐旁开4寸。
9. 中脘：前正中线，脐上4寸。
10. 上脘：脐上6寸。
11. 下脘：脐上2寸。
12. 滑肉门：脐上1寸，旁开2寸。
13. 大包：侧胸部，腋中线上，平第六肋间隙。
14. 天枢：脐旁2寸。
15. 归来：脐下4寸，旁开4寸。
16. 左腹结：在下腹部左侧，脐下1.3寸，旁开4寸。
17. 气海：脐下1.5寸。
18. 关元：脐下3寸。
19. 维道：侧腹部，髂前上棘前下方。
20. 气冲：脐下5寸，旁开2寸。
21. 带脉：侧腹部，第十一肋游离端下方垂线与脐水平线交点。

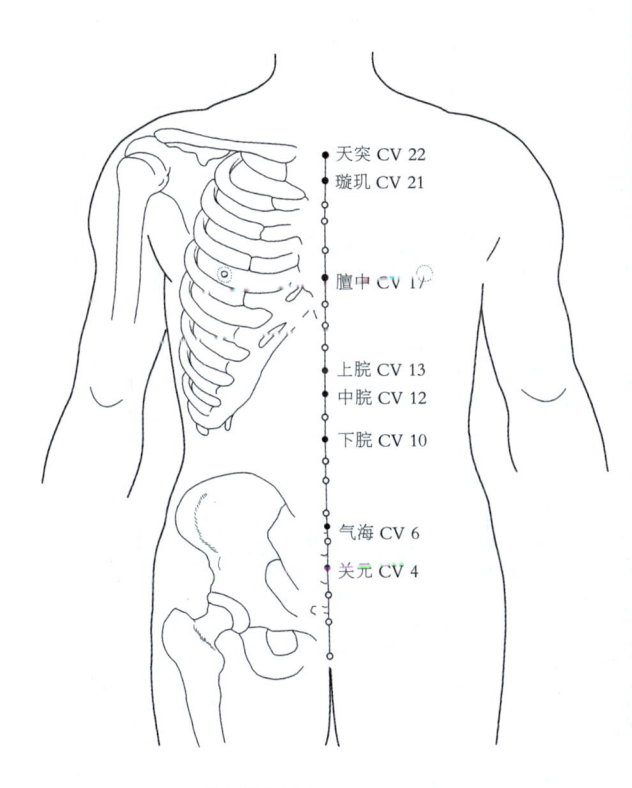

第四章 刮痧疗法常用的部位与穴位
Chapter 4 Common Body Parts and Points Used in Guasha Therapy

- 天突 CV 22
- 璇玑 CV 21
- 膻中 CV 17
- 上脘 CV 13
- 中脘 CV 12
- 下脘 CV 10
- 气海 CV 6
- 关元 CV 4

图33 胸腹部穴位(1)
Fig.33 Points on the chest and abdomen (1)

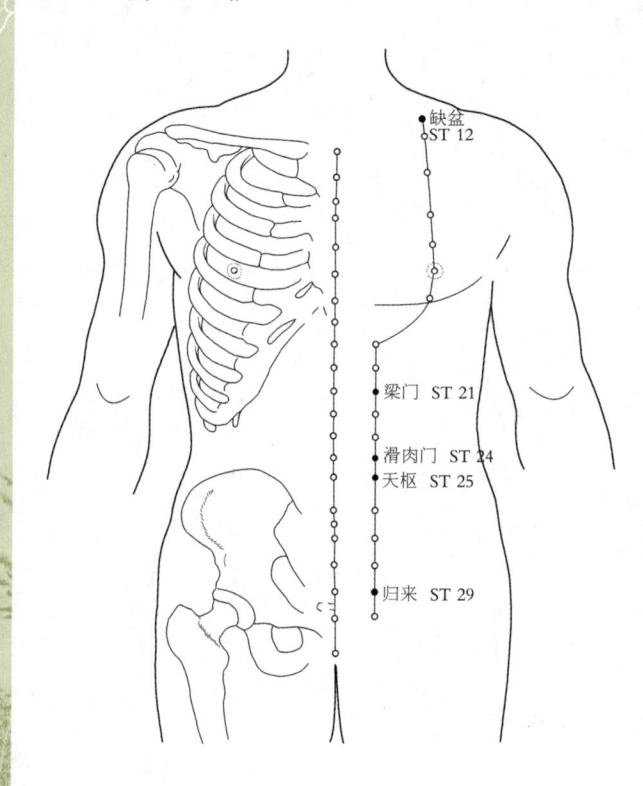

上篇　刮痧疗法的基础理论
Part A　Essential Theory of Guasha Therapy

缺盆
ST 12

梁门　ST 21

滑肉门　ST 24
天枢　ST 25

归来　ST 29

图34　胸腹部穴位(2)
Fig.34 Points on the chest and abdomen (2)

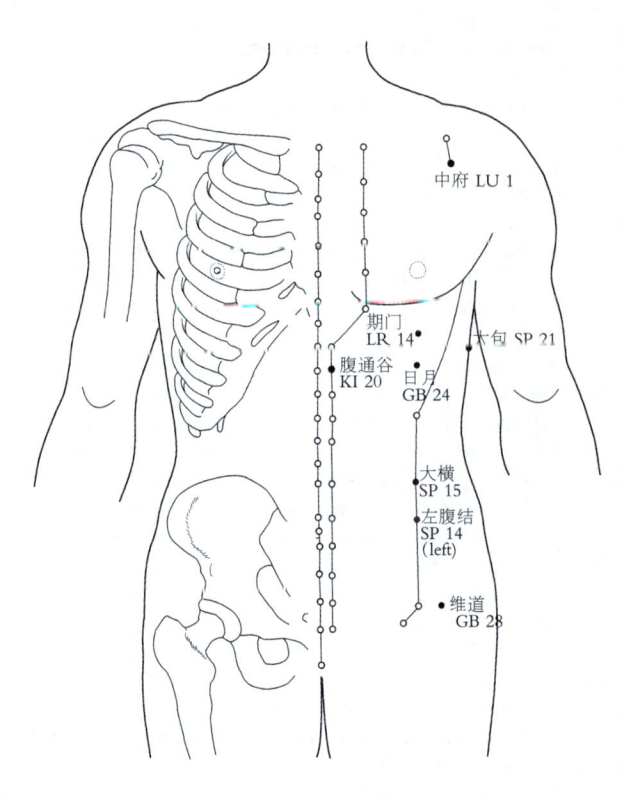

第四章 刮痧疗法常用的部位与穴位
Chapter 4 Common Body Parts and Points Used in Guasha Therapy

中府 LU 1
期门 LR 14
大包 SP 21
腹通谷 KI 20
日月 GB 24
大横 SP 15
左腹结 SP 14 (left)
维道 GB 28

图35 胸腹部穴位(3)
Fig.35 Points on the chest and abdomen (3)

Section 4 Chest and abdomen

(See Fig. 33-35)

1. Tiantu (CV 22): Located in the depression of the suprasternal fossa.

2. Danzhong (CV 17): Located on the anterior midline, level with the 4th intercostal space.

3. Xuanji (CV 21): Located 1 cun below Tiantu (CV 22).

4. Zhongfu (LU 1): Located 6 cun lateral to the anterior midline, at the same level of the 1st intercostal space.

5. Qimen (LR 14): Located directly below the nipple, level with the 6th intercostal space.

6. Liangmen (ST 21): Located 4 cun above the umbilicus, 2 cun lateral to the anterior midline.

7. Futonggu (KI 20): Located 5 cun above the umbilicus, 0.5 cun lateral to the anterior midline.

8. Daheng (SP 15): Located 4 cun lateral to the umbilicus.

9. Zhongwan (CV 12): Located 4 cun above the umbilicus.

10. Shangwan (CV 13): Located 6 cun above the umbilicus.

11. Xiawan (CV 10): Located 2 cun above the umbilicus.

12. Huaroumen (ST 24): Located 1 cun below the umbilicus, 2 cun lateral to the anterior midline.

13. Dabao (SP 21): Located on the mid-axillary line, level with the 6th intercostal space.

14. Tianshu (ST 25): Located 2 cun lateral to the umbilicus.

15. Guilai (ST 29): Located 4 cun below the umbilicus and 4 cun lateral to the anterior midline.

16. Left-sided Fujie (SP 14): Located in the lower abdomen, 1.3 cun below the umbilicus, 4 cun lateral to the frontal midline.

17. Qihai (CV 6): Located 1.5 cun below the umbilicus.

18. Guanyuan (CV 4): Located 3 cun below the umbilicus.
19. Weidao (GB 28): Located immediately anterior and inferior to the anterior superior iliac spine.
20. Qichong (ST 30): Located 5 cun below the umbilicus, 2 cun lateral to the anterior midline.
21. Daimai (GB 26): Located at the intersection of the vertical line directly inferior to the end of the 11th rib and horizontal line of the umbilicus.

第五节　四肢与穴位

（图36～40）

1. 肩髃：上肢外展，肩峰前下方凹陷处。

2. 肩髎：上肢外展，肩髃后方，肩峰后下方呈凹陷处。

3. 肩贞：肩部，腋后横纹上1寸处。

4. 臑俞：肩髎穴下3寸，三角肌的后下方。

5. 肩内陵：肩前，腋前横纹上1寸。

6. 臂臑：肩部，三角肌的下缘。

7. 天府：臂内侧面，腋前横纹头下3寸。

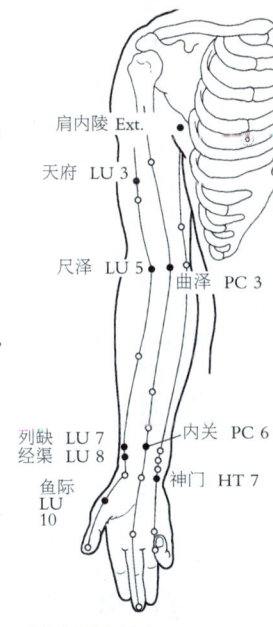

图36 上肢部穴位（1）
Fig.36 Points in the upper extremities (1)

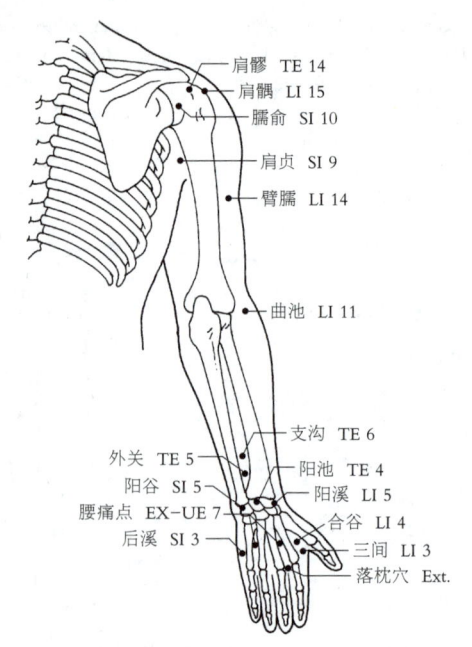

肩髎 TE 14
肩髃 LI 15
臑俞 SI 10
肩贞 SI 9
臂臑 LI 14
曲池 LI 11
支沟 TE 6
外关 TE 5
阳池 TE 4
阳谷 SI 5
阳溪 LI 5
腰痛点 EX-UE 7
合谷 LI 4
后溪 SI 3
三间 LI 3
落枕穴 Ext.

图37 上肢部穴位(2)
Fig.37 Points in the upper extremities (2)

8. 曲泽：肘横纹中，肌腱的尺侧缘。
9. 曲池：屈肘，肘横纹头与肱骨外上髁连线中点。
10. 肘髎：手臂外侧，曲池穴上1寸。
11. 尺泽：肘横纹中，肱二头肌肌腱的桡侧缘。

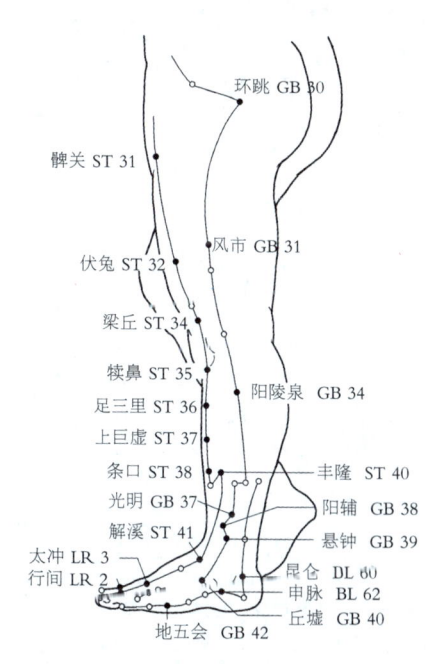

第四章 刮痧疗法常用的部位与穴位
Chapter 4 Common Body Parts and Points Used in Guasha Therapy

环跳 GB 30
髀关 ST 31
风市 GB 31
伏兔 ST 32
梁丘 ST 34
犊鼻 ST 35
阳陵泉 GB 34
足三里 ST 36
上巨虚 ST 37
条口 ST 38
丰隆 ST 40
光明 GB 37
阳辅 GB 38
解溪 ST 41
悬钟 GB 39
太冲 LR 3
昆仑 BL 60
行间 LR 2
申脉 BL 62
丘墟 GB 40
地五会 GB 42

图38 下肢穴位（1）
Fig.38 Points in lower extremities (1)

12. 内关：腕横纹上2寸，两筋之间。

13. 外关：腕背横纹上2寸，两骨之间。

14. 列缺：腕关节，桡骨茎突上方，腕横纹上1.5寸。

15. 鱼际：掌侧，第一掌骨中点，赤白肉际之间。

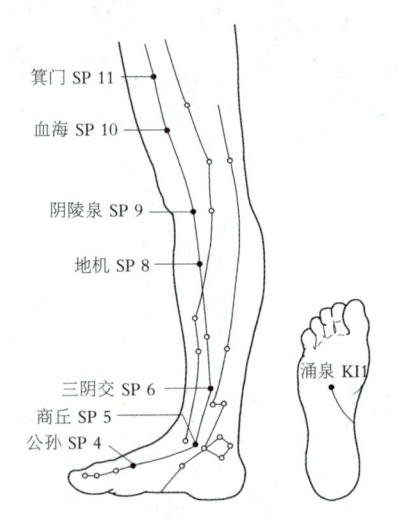

箕门 SP 11
血海 SP 10
阴陵泉 SP 9
地机 SP 8
三阴交 SP 6
商丘 SP 5
公孙 SP 4
涌泉 KI1

图39 下肢穴位(2)
Fig. 39 Points in lower extremities (2)

16. 经渠：掌侧，腕横纹上1寸，动脉桡侧。
17. 支沟：腕背横纹上3寸，两骨之间凹陷处。
18. 神门：腕掌侧横纹尺侧端，肌腱的桡侧凹陷。
19. 阳池：腕背横纹桡侧，两筋之间凹陷处。
20. 阳溪：腕背横纹上，拇指上翘两筋之间。
21. 阳谷：手腕尺侧，尺骨茎突与三角骨之间的凹陷处。
22. 四缝：第二至第五指掌侧近端指关节的中央。（图119）
23. 腰痛点：手背侧，第二、第三掌骨及第四、第五掌骨之间，腕横纹与掌指关节中点。

24. 三间：第二掌指关节小头后凹陷处。

25. 后溪：第五掌指关节小头后下方，赤白肉际之间。

26. 合谷：虎口处，近第二掌骨中点处。

27. 十宣：十指末端。

28. 落枕穴：第二、第三掌指关节小头后凹陷处。

29. 环跳：侧卧屈股，股骨大转子高点与骶管裂孔连线的外1/3与内2/3交点处。

30. 承扶：臀横纹的中点。

31. 髀关：大腿前面，髂前上棘与髌底外侧端连线上，屈股平会阴。

32. 伏兔：大腿前面，髂前上棘与髌底外侧端连线上，髌底上6寸。

33. 箕门：大腿内侧，髌骨内上角上8寸。

34. 风市：大腿外侧部中线，直立垂手时，中指尖处。

35. 殷门：承扶穴下6寸。

36. 梁丘：屈膝，髌底外侧端上2寸。

37. 血海：大腿内侧，髌底内侧端上2寸。

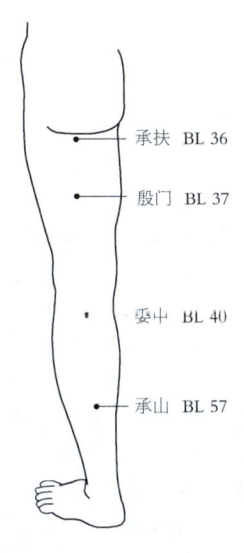

承扶 BL 36
殷门 BL 37
委中 BL 40
承山 BL 57

图40 下肢穴位（3）
Fig.40 Points in lower extremities (3)

38. 委中：膝后腘窝正中。

39. 阴陵泉：小腿内侧，当胫骨内侧髁后下方凹陷处。

40. 足三里：膝盖下外侧凹陷下3寸，距胫骨前缘外1横指。

41. 丰隆：足三里下5寸，旁开1横指。

42. 上巨虚：足三里下3寸。

43. 条口：足三里下5寸。

44. 地机：阴陵泉下3寸。

45. 阳辅：外踝尖上4寸，腓骨前缘稍前方。

46. 三阴交：足内踝尖上3寸，胫骨内侧缘后方。

47. 悬钟：外踝高点上3寸，腓骨前缘。

48. 阳陵泉：小腿外侧，腓骨小头前下方凹陷处。

49. 膝眼：髌韧带两侧凹陷处。

50. 承山：小腿后侧，当伸膝或提足跟时，腓肠肌肌腹出现尖角凹陷处。

51. 丘墟：足外踝前下方凹陷中。

52. 商丘：足内踝前下方凹陷中。

53. 昆仑：外踝尖与跟腱之间连线中点。

54. 解溪：足背与小腿交界处的横纹中央，两筋之间凹陷处。

55. 公孙：足内侧缘，第一跖骨基底的前下方。

56. 申脉：外踝高点下凹陷处。

57. 光明：外踝尖上5寸，腓骨前缘。

58. 地五会：足背外侧，第四跖趾关节的后方。

59. 行间：足背第一、第二趾间缝纹端。

60. 太溪：内踝尖与跟腱之间凹陷处。

61. 太冲：足背侧，第一跖骨间隙后方凹陷处。

62. 涌泉：足底人字沟顶点。

Section 5 Four extremities

(See Fig. 36-40)

1. Jianyu (LI 15): Located in the depression anterior and inferior to the acromion when the arm is in full abduction.

2. Jianliao (SJ 14): Located in the depression posterior and inferior to the acromion when the arm is in full abduction, approximately 1 cun posterior to Jianyu (LI 15).

3. Jianzhen (SI 9): Located 1 cun above the posterior end of the axillary fold when the arm is abducted.

4. Naoshu (SI 10): Located 3 cun below Jianliao (SJ 14), posterior and inferior to the deltoid muscle.

5. Jianneiling (also known as Jianqian) (Extra): Located 1 cun above the anterior axillary fold.

6. Binao (LI 14): Located on the radial side of the humerus, superior to the lower border of the deltoid muscle.

7. Tianfu (LU 3): Located on the medial aspect of the upper arm, 3 cun below the end of axillary fold.

8. Quze (PC 3): Located on the transverse cubital crease, on the ulnar side of the tendon of biceps brachii muscle.

9. Quchi (LI 11): Located on a line, midway between the end of transverse cubital crease and lateral condyle of the humerus when the elbow is flexed.

10. Zhouliao (LI 12): Located on the lateral aspect of the arm, 1 cun superolateral to Quchi (LI 11).

11. Chize (LU 5): Located on the transverse cubital crease, on the

radial side of the tendon of biceps brachii muscle.

12. **Neiguan (PC 6)**: Located 2 cun above the transverse crease of the wrist, between the two tendons.

13. **Waiguan (SJ 5)**: Located 2 cun above the transverse crease of the dorsum of the wrist, between the radius and ulna.

14. **Lieque (LU 7)**: Located at superior to the styloid process, 1.5 cun above the transverse crease of the wrist.

15. **Yuji (LU 10)**: Located on the radial aspect of the midpoint of the first metacarpal bone, on the junction between the red and white skin.

16. **Jingqu (LU 8)**: Located 1 cun above the transverse crease of the wrist, in the depression on the lateral side of the radial artery.

17. **Zhigou (SJ 6)**: Located 3 cun above the transverse crease of the he dorsum of the wrist, between radius and ulna.

18. **Shenmen (HT 7)**: Located on the ulnar side of the transverse crease of the wrist, in the depression on the radial side of the tendon of m. flexor carpi ulnaris.

19. **Yangchi (SJ 4)**: Located on the radial side of the transverse crease of the dorsum of the wrist, in a depression between the two tendons.

20. **Yangxi (LI 5)**: Located on the transverse crease of the dorsum of the wrist, in the depression between the two tendons when the thumb is raised.

21. **Yanggu (SI 5)**: Located on the ulnar side of the transverse crease of the dorsum of the wrist, in the depression between the styloid process of the ulna and the triquetral bone.

22. **Sifeng (EX-UE 10)**: Located at the midpoint of the transverse crease of the proximal interphalangeal joints of the index, ring, and little fingers. (See Fig. 119)

23. Yaotongdian (EX-UE 7): Located on the dorsum of the hand, between the 2nd and 3rd metacarpal bones, and the 4th and 5th metacarpal bones. In total, 4 points on both hands.

24. Sanjian (LI 3): Located in the depression proximal to the head of the 2nd metacarpal bone.

25. Houxi (SI 3): Located posterior and inferior to the head of 5th metacarpophalangeal joint, at the junction between the red and white skin.

26. Hegu (LI 4): Located between the 1st and 2nd metacarpal bones, approximately in the center of the 2nd metacarpal bone on the radial side.

27. Shixuan (EX-UE 11): Located at the tips of the ten fingers.

28. Luozhenxue (Extra): Located in the depression posterior to the head of 2nd and 3rd metacarpophalangeal joints.

29. Huantiao (GB 30): Located on a line from the great trochanter to the hiatus of sacrum when the patient take a side lying position with the thigh flexed.

30. Chengfu (BL 36): Located in the middle of the transverse gluteal fold.

31. Biguan (ST 31): Located on the line connecting the anterior superior iliac spine and lateral border of the patella, at the same level of perineum when the thigh is flexed.

32. Futu (ST 32): Located on the line connecting the anterior superior iliac spine and lateral border of the patella, 6 cun above the base of the patella.

33. Jimen (SP 11): Located 8 cun above the mediosuperior border of the patella.

34. Fengshi (GB 31): Located on the midline of the lateral aspect of the thigh. When the patient is standing erect with the hands close by

the sides, the point is where the tip of the middle finger touches the thigh.

35. Yinmen (BL 37): Located 6 cun below Chengfu (BL 36).

36. Liangqiu (ST 34): Located 2 cun above the laterosuperior border of the patella when the knee is flexed.

37. Xuehai (SP 10): Located 2 cun above the mediosuperior border of the patella.

38. Weizhong (BL 40): Located at the midpoint of the transverse crease of the popliteal fossa.

39. Yinlingquan (SP 9): Located in the depression posterior and inferior to the medial condyle of the tibia.

40. Zusanli (ST 36): Located 3 cun below the depression of the lateral end of patellar ligament, 1 finger-breadth from the anterior crest of the tibia.

41. Fenglong (ST 40): Located 5 cun below Zusanli (ST 36), 1 finger-breadth lateral to Tiaokou (ST 38).

42. Shangjuxu (ST 37): Located 3 cun below Zusanli (ST 36).

43. Tiaokou (ST 38): Located 5 cun below Zusanli (ST 36).

44. Diji (SP 8): Located 3 cun below Yinlingquan (SP 9).

45. Yangfu (GB 38): Located 4 cun above the tip of the lateral malleolus, slightly anterior to the anterior border of the fibula.

46. Sanyinjiao (SP 6): Located 3 cun directly above the tip of the medial malleolus, on the posterior border of the medial aspect of the tibia.

47. Xuanzhong (GB 39): Located 3 cun above the tip of the lateral malleolus, on the anterior border of the fibula.

48. Yanglingquan (GB 34): Located in the depression anterior and inferior to the head of the fibula.

49. Xiyan (ST 35): Located in the two depressions bilateral to the

patellar ligament (2 points).

50. Chengshan (BL 57): Located directly below the belly of gastrocnemius muscle when the knee is extended or heel is lifted.

51. Qiuxu (GB 40): Located in the depression anterior and inferior to the lateral malleolus.

52. Shangqiu (SP 5): Located in the depression distal and inferior to the medial malleolus.

53. Kunlun (BL 60): Located at the midpoint of the line connecting the tip of external malleolus and Achilles tendon.

54. Jiexi (ST 41): Located at the midpoint of the transverse crease of the ankle joint, in the depression between the two tendons.

55. Gongsun (SP 4): Located in the depression distal and inferior to the base of the 1st metatarsal bone, at the junction of the red and white skin.

56. Shenmai (BL 62): Located in the depression directly below the lateral malleolus.

57. Guangming (GB 37): Located 5 cun directly above the tip of the external malleolus, on the anterior border of the fibula.

58. Diwuhui (GB 42): Located on the lateral side of the foot dorsum, posterior to the 4th metatarsal bone.

59. Xingjian (LR 2): Located on the dorsum of the foot, between the 1st and 2nd toes, proximal to the margin of the web.

60. Taixi (KI 3): Located in the depression between the tip of medial malleolus and Achilles tendon.

61. Taichong (LR 3): Located on the dorsum of the foot, in the depression posterior to the heads of the first metatarsal bone.

62. Yongquan (KI 1): Located approximately at the junction of the anterior 1/3 and posterior 2/3 of the sole of the foot.

附：皮部分布图
Attached: Profile of cutaneous regions

【注】1.任脉皮部；2.手阳明大肠经皮部；3.手太阴肺经皮部；4.手厥阴心包经皮部；5.手少阴心经皮部；6.足少阳胆经皮部；7.足少阴肾经皮部；8.足厥阴肝经皮部；9.足太阴脾经皮部；10.足阳明胃经皮部。（图41）

Remark: The cutaneous regions of: 1. The Conception Vessel; 2. The large intestine meridian; 3. The lung meridian; 4. The pericardium

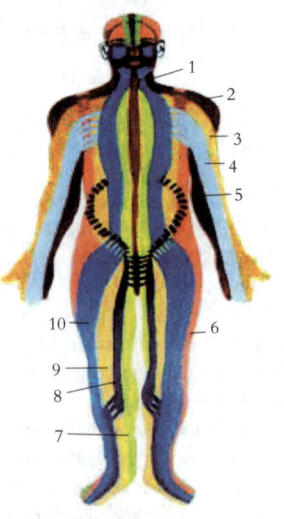

图41 皮部分布图—正面观
Fig.41 Profile of cutaneous regions-front view

meridian; 5. The heart meridian; 6. The gallbladder meridian; 7. The kidney meridian; 8. The liver meridian; 9. the spleen meridian; 10. The stomach meridian. (See Fig. 41)

【注】1.任脉皮部；2.足少阴肾经皮部；3.足阳明胃经皮部；4.足太阴脾经皮部；5.足太阳膀胱经皮部；6.足少阳胆经皮部；7.手阳明大肠经皮部；8.手少阳三焦经皮部；9.手太阳小肠经皮部。（图42）

Remark: The cutaneous regions of: 1. The Conception Vessel; 2. The kidney meridian; 3. The stomach meridian; 4. The spleen

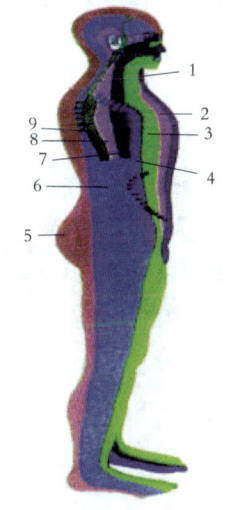

图42 皮部分布图—侧面观
Fig.42 Profile of cutaneous regions–side view

meridian; 5. The bladder meridian; 6. The gallbladder meridian; 7. The large intestine meridian; 8. The Sanjiao meridian; 9. The small intestine meridian. (See Fig. 42)

【注】1.督脉皮部；2.手阳明大肠经皮部；3.手少阳三焦经皮部；4.手太阳小肠经皮部；5.足太阳膀胱经皮部；6.足少阳胆经皮部。（图43）

Remark: The cutaneous regions of : 1. The Governor Vessel; 2. The large intestine meridian; 3. The Sanjiao meridian; 4. The small intestine meridian; 5. The bladder meridian; 6. The gallbladder meridian. (See Fig. 43)

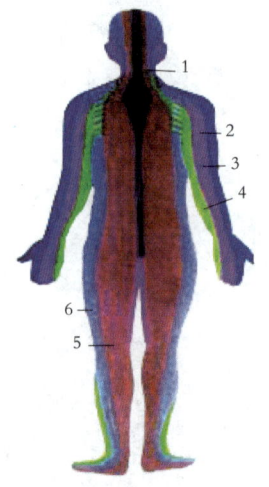

图43 皮部分布图—背面观
Fig.43 Profile of cutaneous regions–back view

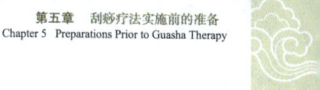

第五章　刮痧疗法实施前的准备

在实施刮痧疗法之前必须做好相应的准备。在选穴上，刮痧选穴配穴的原则是以中医的脏腑经络理论为指导，根据临床病症的不同进行辨证施治，并结合腧穴的功能、特性进行配穴。另外，选择适当的刮痧体位也尤为重要。

第一节　选穴原则

1. 近部选穴原则：又称局部取穴原则。即是在病变的局部或邻近的部位选取穴位进行治疗的原则。具有驱除局部邪气、疏通患处经脉气血、消瘀止痛等作用。多用于治疗病变脏腑、器官、经脉、经筋、四肢、关节、韧带等部位的病痛。临床上对于跌仆、扭挫伤、痛证等常取压痛点（又称"阿是穴"），即属于此类选穴范畴。

2. 远部选穴原则：又称远道取穴原则。即是选取远离病变部位的穴位进行治疗。如咽喉肿痛，取鱼际、太溪；胃痛，取足三里、内关；牙痛，取合谷、内庭等都属于此类选穴范畴。

3. 随证选穴原则：又称辨证或对证选穴原则。它是针对一些病变部位不明确或全身性的疾病，需结合腧穴的特殊作用而设的一种选穴原则。如发热，取大椎、曲池；高血压，取涌泉、太溪等。

Chapter 5 Preparations Prior to Guasha Therapy

Preparing appropriate measures is important prior to commencing Guasha therapy. These preparations usually include the following three aspects: principle of point selection, point combination, and adopting an appropriate body position.

Section 1 Principle of point selection

1. Proximal or local points: These points are located at or adjacent to the affected area and can be used to remove the local pathogenic-qi, activate local qi and blood circulation, resolve stasis and relieve pain. This principle is indicated for pain involving zang-fu organs, meridians, sinews, four extremities, joints, and ligaments. Points of tenderness, also known as Ashi points, are also frequently selected for traumatic injuries, sprains or contusions, and pain syndrome.

2. Distal points: These points are located far from the affected area. For example, the points Yuji (LU 10) and Taixi (KI 3) can be selected for sore throat; Zusanli (ST 36) and Neiguan (PC 6) for gastric pain; and Hegu (LI 4) and Neiting (ST 44) for toothache.

3. Points selected on the basis of pattern identification: These points are usually selected for unspecific disease locations or systemic disorders. For example, Dazhui (GV 14) and Quchi (LI 11) can be selected for fever, and Yongquan (KI 1) and Taixi (KI 3) for hypertension.

第二节 配穴方法

1. **本经配穴法**：在确定某一脏腑经脉发生病变时，选取该脏腑经脉的腧穴进行配伍。如咳嗽，取肺经的中府、尺泽、太渊等。

2. **表里经配穴法**：依据人体的脏腑经脉具有相互表里络属的关系，脏腑经脉之间在生理上互相依存，在病变时互相影响的特性而定，即肺与大肠、心与小肠、脾与胃、肝与胆、肾与膀胱。如胃痛，可以取胃经的穴位中脘、足三里、梁丘等，也可以结合取脾经的地机、阴陵泉等。

3. **上下配穴法**：即选取人体腰以上部位的穴位和腰以下部位的穴位配伍治疗疾病的方法。如颈椎病，上可取颈部的风池、大椎等，下可取腰骶部、下肢的肾俞、昆仑等。

4. **前后配穴法**：又称"腹背阴阳配穴法"。即取胸腹部的穴位和腰背部的穴位相互配伍应用。多用于治疗脏腑的病变。如咳嗽、哮喘，前取中府、膻中等，后取肺俞、风门、膏肓等。

5. **左右配穴法**：根据经脉循行有左右交叉的原理，即在配穴时可左病取右或右病取左。如一侧的腰痛，可取对侧的腰眼、肾俞或取双侧。此法对于中风偏瘫或疼痛性疾病，如扭伤等有良好的效果。

6. **远近配穴法**：即选取病变的局部、邻近部位或远隔部位的穴位配伍应用。如牙痛近取颊车、下关等，远取合谷、太溪等。

7. **辨证配穴法**：在中医辨证施治的原则指导下，根据病变的病因、病机，结合操作者的临床经验进行配穴应用。如咳嗽，因感受风寒引起，取风门、列缺；因胃肠道功能低下、脾虚生痰引起，取中府、肺俞、足三里等；因恼怒肝郁肝火引起，取膻中、期门、支沟等。这种方法实际上是以上各种方法的综合应用。

以上各种配穴方法，除了某些疾病的特殊需要外，一般每次选穴以2～5个穴位为宜。

Section 2　Method of point combination

1. Point combination on a single meridian: For pathologic changes in the meridian of a specific zang or fu organ, select points in the same meridian, for example, the lung points Zhongfu (LU 1), Chize (LU 5), and Taiyuan (LU 9) can be combined to treat cough.

2. Point combination on the interior-exterior related meridians: Since zang-fu organs may depend on each other physiologically and interact with each other pathologically through the interior-exterior meridian relationship, point combination of these related meridians can be effective, for example, the stomach points Zusanli (ST 36) and Liangqiu (ST 34) and the spleen points Diji (SP 8) and Yinlingquan (SP 9) can be combined for gastric pain. Similarly, relationships exist between the lung and large intestine, heart and small intestine, liver and gallbladder, and kidney and bladder.

3. Upper and lower body point combination: The points above or below the lumbar region can be combined to treat disorders, for example, the upper body points Fengchi (GB 20) and Dazhui (GV 14) and the lower body points Shenshu (BL 23) and Kunlun (BL 60) can be combined for cervical spondylosis.

4. Posterior and anterior point combination (also known as abdomen-back or yin-yang point combination): For example, the points on the chest, Zhongfu (LU 1) and Danzhong (CV 17) and points on the back, Feishu (BL 13), Fengmen (BL 12), and Gaohuang (BL

43) can be combined to treat cough and asthma.

5. Left and right point combination: Since meridians may cross from one side of the body to the other, sometimes the points in the left side can be selected to treat problems on the right side or vice versa. For example, the contralateral or bilateral Yaoyan (EX-B 7) and Shenshu (BL 23) can be selected for one-side low back pain. This principle is especially helpful for hemiplegia after stroke or pain due to sprain.

6. Distal and proximal point combination: The points adjacent to or distal to affected areas can be combined to treat some conditions. For example, the proximal points Jiache (ST 6) and Xiaguan (ST 7) and the distal points Hegu (LI 4) and Taixi (KI 3) can be combined to treat toothache.

7. Point combination based on pattern identification: On the basis of analysis of the etiological and pathogenic factors according to TCM theory as well as personal experience, some points can be combined to treat certain conditions. For example, the points Fengmen (BL 12) and Lieque (LU 7) can be selected to treat cough due to wind-cold; the points Zhongfu (LU 1), Feishu (BL 13), and Zusanli (ST 36) can be selected to treat cough due to spleen deficiency related to phlegm; and the points Danzhong (CV 17), Qimen (LR 14), and Zhigou (SJ 6) can be selected for cough due to liver-qi stagnation transforming into fire.

Except in specific cases, 2-5 points are selected each time.

第三节　刮痧患者体位的选择

一般而言，刮痧的体位是以刮痧时施术者能确定刮拭部位、便于操作、患者舒适又能充分暴露刮治部位为原则。在可能的情况下，尽量采用一种体位完成全部治疗方案。对于体弱或精神过度紧张者，应采用卧位施术。常用的体位有：

一、卧位

1. 俯卧位：适宜于头项、背腰及臀、下肢的刮拭。（图44）
2. 侧卧位：适宜于身体侧面或上下肢的刮拭。（图45）
3. 仰卧位：适宜于头面、胸腹部以及四肢部的刮拭。（图46）

二、坐位

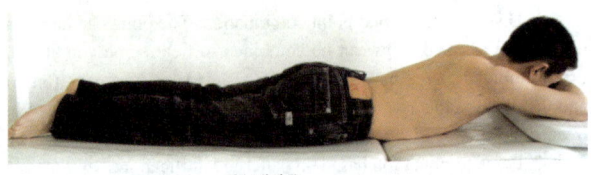

图44 俯卧位
Fig.44 A prone position

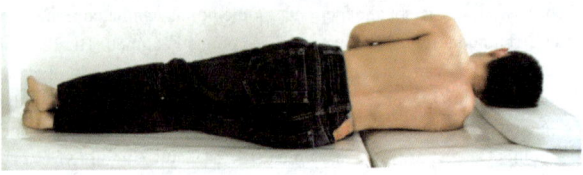

图45 侧卧位
Fig.45 A side-lying position

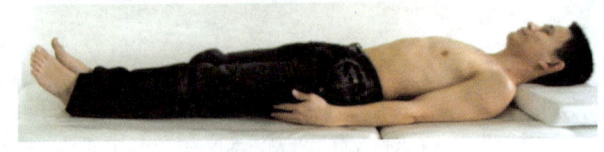

图46 仰卧位
Fig.46 A supine position

1. **俯伏坐位**：适宜于后头、肩项、背部、上肢的刮拭。（图47）
2. **侧伏坐位**：适宜于头部一侧、面颊、耳前后、颈项、一侧肩及上肢的刮拭。（图48）
3. **仰靠坐位**：适宜于前头、颜面、颈部、胸部、上肢或膝以下部位的刮拭。（图49）

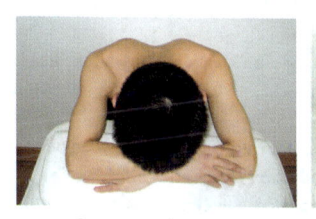

图47 俯伏坐位
Fig.47 A prone sitting position

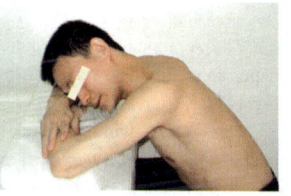

图48 侧伏坐位
Fig.48 A lateral prone sitting position

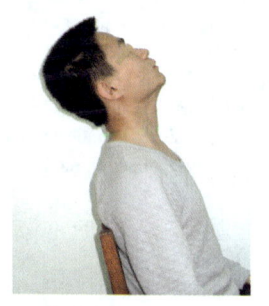

图49 仰靠坐位
Fig.49 A supine sitting position

Section 3 Selection of body position

Generally the patients should adopt a comfortable position to fully expose the area to be treated and enable the practitioner to operate conveniently. It is strongly advised to complete the whole procedure with one position. In addition, those with a weak constitution or excessive nervousness should adopt a lying position. The common positions are as follows:

1. Lying position

1.1 A prone position is indicated for Guasha therapy on the head, nape, upper back, lower back, buttocks, and lower extremities. (See Fig.44)

1.2 A side-lying position is indicated for Guasha therapy on lateral side of the body or upper and lower extremities. (See Fig.45)

1.3 A supine position is indicated for Guasha therapy on the head, face, abdomen, chest, and four extremities. (See Fig.46)

2. Sitting position

2.1 A prone sitting position is indicated for Guasha therapy on the occipit, shoulder, nape, back, and upper extremities. (See Fig.47)

2.2 A lateral prone sitting position is indicated for Guasha therapy on one-sided head, cheek, auricular area, neck and nape, one-sided shoulder, and upper extremities. (See Fig.48)

2.3 A supine sitting position is indicated for Guasha therapy on the forehead, face, neck, chest, upper extremities, and areas below the knee. (See Fig.49)

第六章 刮痧疗法的操作方法

第一节 施术前的操作

1. 检查刮痧用具，尤其是刮痧板的边缘，应光滑、完好，刮痧板应富有弹性。
2. 选择好受试者的体位，并暴露需刮拭的部位。
3. 用热毛巾蘸肥皂将准备刮痧的部位擦拭干净，或用75%乙醇局部常规消毒。
4. 在刮痧部位涂抹适当的刮痧介质。（图50）

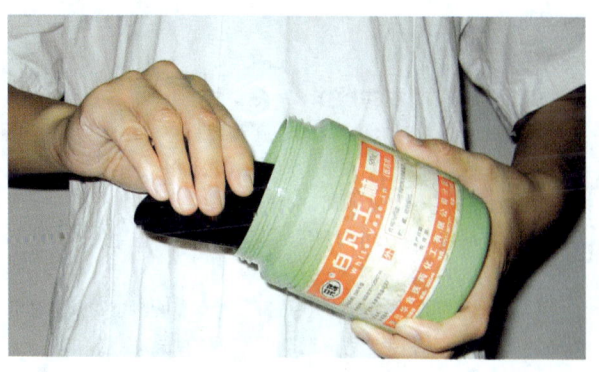

图50 施术前涂凡士林
Fig.50 Applying Vaseline prior to Guasha therapy

Chapter 6　Operational Procedures of Guasha Therapy

Section 1 Procedures prior to Guasha therapy

1. Check the Guasha tools, particularly the edge of the Guasha board: the edge should be smooth and intact; and the board should be elastic.

2. Help the patient adopt an appropriate body position to fully expose the area to be treated.

3. Clean the areas to be treated with a warm towel soaked in soapy water or do local routine sterilization with 75% alcohol.

4. Apply an appropriate Guasha medium in the area to be treated. (See Fig.50)

第二节　施术中的操作

1. 施术者以右手拿刮痧工具，用腕力和臂力，力度要适当，由轻开始，逐渐加重。动作节奏均匀，以受试者能耐受为度，刮拭除特殊要求外，一般要求将刮拭范围拉长。

2. 刮痧时应顺一个方向刮拭，自上而下、自内而外，井然有序。

3. 常见的刮拭顺序依次为头颈部、背部、胸腹、四肢。对于体弱、久病、小儿和年老者应选择相对较轻的手法。

4. 一般刮10～20次或15～20分钟，以出现紫红色斑点或斑块为度。（图51）

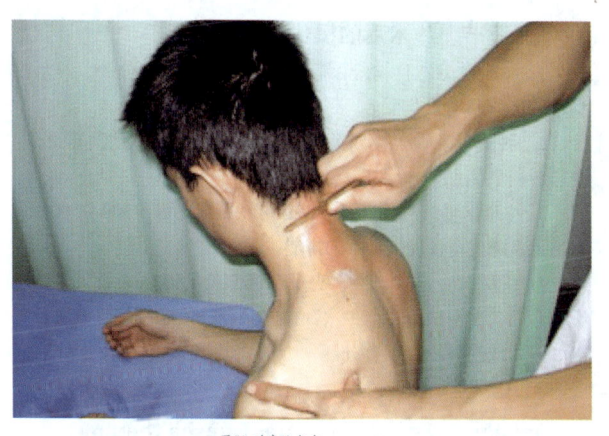

图51 刮痧施术中
Fig.51 during Guasha therapy

Section 2 Procedures during Guasha therapy

1. Holding the Guasha tool by the right hand, the practitioner should use gradually increasing but tolerable force, from the wrist and arm, with an even rhythm. Except for special requirements, the range of each scrape should be long

2. Scrape in one direction, from upward to downward or from inward to outward.

3. The common order for scraping is: head, neck, back, chest, abdomen, and the four extremities. Mild force is advised for children, the elderly, and those with a weak constitution or a chronic condition.

4. One Guasha treatment usually lasts 10-20 strokes or for about 15-20 minutes until purple red spots or petechia appear. (See Fig.51)

第三节 施术后的操作

1. 一般在患者自觉轻松后,可让其休息2~3分钟,然后在刮过的部位刮动十几下。

2. 刮拭结束时,应以消毒棉球或干净绵纸揩拭刮拭部位,令患者稍事休息。

3. 注意保暖,避免迎风着凉,可饮服温开水(300~500ml),以增强新陈代谢,促进毒素的排泄。

4. 在刮拭后1~2天内,出现刮痧部位的疼痛一般属于正常反应,第二次刮拭应在前一次刮拭的痧点(紫红斑点或斑块)基本消失后或间隔3~5天后进行。

Section 3 Procedures after Guasha therapy

1. Ask the patient to rest for 2-3 minutes after they feel relaxed, then tap the scraped area many times.

2. Wipe or clean the scraped area with aseptic cotton ball or dry tissue paper after the Guasha is complete and ask the patient to rest for a while.

3. Tell the patient to keep warm and avoid wind attack. Ask the patient to drink warm water (300-500 ml) to promote metabolism and discharge of toxins.

4. The patient may experience pain (normal reaction) on the scraped area within 1-2 days. The next Guasha treatment should start after the disappearance of purple red spots or petechia or 3-5 days after the first treatment.

第七章 刮痧疗法的适应证

刮痧疗法具有疏通经络、活血化瘀、开窍泄热、通达阳气、泻秽浊、排毒素等作用。适用于实热或湿热的急性"痧证",也可广泛用于内、外、妇、儿、耳鼻喉科等出现气机痹阻、经络瘀滞,表现为以疼痛、酸胀等为主症,如中暑、发热、感冒、高血压、急性吐泻、急性咽喉肿痛、目赤肿痛、扭挫伤、头痛、腰痛、落枕、顽固性痹证、消化不良、痛经等急慢性疾患。

Chapter 7 Indications for Guasha Therapy

The Guasha therapy acts to dredge meridians and activate blood circulation to resolve stasis. It opens orifices, clears heat, discharges turbidity, and removes toxins. It is indicated for acute 'Sha syndrome' due to excessive or deficient heat. It is also indicated for general conditions of internal medicine, external medicine, gynecology, pediatrics, and ear-nose-throat problems that manifest as pain, soreness, and distension due to qi stagnation of the meridians. These conditions include sunstroke, fever, common cold, hypertension, acute vomiting and diarrhea, acute sore throat, conjunctivitis, sprain or contusion, headache, lower back pain, stiff neck, intractable bi-impediment syndrome, dyspepsia, and dysmenorrhea.

第八章 刮痧疗法的禁忌证与注意事项

一、禁忌证

1. **疾病禁忌**：各种急慢性传染病、急性高热不退、急性骨髓炎、结核性关节炎、急腹症或传染性皮肤病、糖尿病、出血性疾病如血小板减少症或凝血功能障碍的患者，刮痧疗法则不宜使用。

2. **部位禁忌**：各种皮肤溃疡、疮疡、烫伤等及患者新近骨折或伤口部位，不宜应用刮痧疗法。

3. **穴位禁忌**：行经期、妊娠期妇女的腰骶部及身体的一些穴位更禁止应用，如三阴交、合谷、肩井、昆仑等。否则，可能导致经期紊乱、流产或早产。

4. **生理禁忌**：妇女的"四期"，即行经期、妊娠期、哺乳期、更年期应慎用刮痧疗法。过饥、过饱、过劳或过度紧张的患者应慎用或暂时不进行刮痧。

二、注意事项

1. 小儿、年老体弱、久病体虚、有严重心脑血管疾病等患者，应慎用。即使施用，也应轻刮或隔衣刮拭，并让患者选择舒适的体位。

2. 操作前应注意操作室内的温度和通风情况，注意保暖、保持空气流通。

3. 在实施过程中应避免用力过猛或用力不均、节奏不一、次序无章。

4. 实施的时间应以每次每个部位刮拭不超过10分钟为宜，或以出痧为度，而不应强求。

5. 个别患者在刮拭过程中出现面色苍白、胸闷恶心、出冷汗等的"晕刮"现象，应停止操作，予以平卧，服用加糖的热开水，稍事休息即可好转，也可按压水沟、内关等穴位。

6. 每次刮痧结束后，应嘱患者休息片刻，避免即刻迎风劳作或冲凉。禁食生冷、油腻或难以消化的食物。

7. 用于强身保健的刮痧，应以轻手法或采用隔衣刮痧法，刮拭部位不强求出现痧痕。

Chapter 8 Precautions for Guasha Therapy

1. Contraindications

1.1 Contraindicated conditions: Various acute or chronic infectious diseases, acute persistent high-grade fever, acute osteomyelitis, tuberculous arthritis, acute abdomen or infectious skin disease, diabetes, and hemorrhagic conditions such as thrombopenia or coagulation disorders.

1.2 Contraindicated body parts: Body parts with skin ulcers, sores, scalding, recent fracture, or wounds.

1.3 Contraindicated points: Points located in the lumbosacral area or special points for women during menstruation or pregnancy, such as Sanyinjiao (SP 6), Hegu (LI 4), Jianjing (GB 21), and Kunlun (BL 60); otherwise, it may cause irregular period, miscarriage, or premature birth.

1.4 Physiological contraindications: During menstruation, pregnancy, lactation, or menopause, and those with excessive hunger, overeat, fatigue or nervousness.

2. Cautionary notes

2.1 It is not advisable to use Guasha therapy on small children, the elderly, or those with a weak constitution, chronic conditions or severe cardio-cerebrovascular diseases. In these cases mild Guasha or scraping with clothes in a comfortable body position may be applied.

2.2 Maintain an appropriate room temperature and good ventilation prior to Guasha therapy.

2.3 During the treatment, avoid sudden or uneven force with an irregular rhythm or order.

2.4 Scrape no more than 10 min in each area, or stop on the appearance of red spots (Sha).

2.5 In case of 'Guasha fainting' phenomenon such as a pale complexion, chest stuffiness, nausea, and cold sweats, stop scraping immediately, help the patient to lie flat and drink warm water with sugar. Renzhong (GV 26) and Neiguan (PC 6) can also be pressed. In most cases the patient will feel better after a while.

2.6 Tell the patient to rest for a while after each Guasha treatment to avoid wind and fatigue. Also avoid showering in cold water. Ask the patient to stay away from raw, cold, oily or hard-to-digest food.

2.7 When Guasha is used for health preservation, the practitioner may use mild manipulation or scraping over the clothes. The appearance of red spots or petechia is not necessary.

下篇 刮痧疗法的实践应用
Part B Guasha Therapy in Practice

第九章 内科病症的刮痧疗法应用

第一节 中暑

中暑，俗称"发痧"。夏季多发。轻者表现为突然头昏、头痛、心中烦乱、无汗、恶心、指甲或口唇紫绀。重者出现壮热、烦躁、气短、汗出、四肢厥冷、神昏、抽搐或血压下降、腹部剧痛等。若治疗不及时，易出现高热、昏迷甚至危及生命。

【主穴】大椎、曲池、尺泽、委中。（图52~54）

【配穴】胸闷配膻中；恶心配内关；神昏配水沟；腹痛配中脘；头痛配印堂、太阳、风池；还可配刮脊柱两旁。

【操作方法】

1. 重刮主穴，每穴及其两侧各3行，以出现痧痕为度。

2. 根据出现随症的不同加刮配穴。其中头痛先以手撮印堂至痧痕出现，再推印堂至太阳，最后以刮痧板由太阳刮至风池；水沟以指掐法，用力向鼻根部推挤；天枢配合拔火罐。

3. 也可直接刮脊柱两旁，自上而下轻轻顺

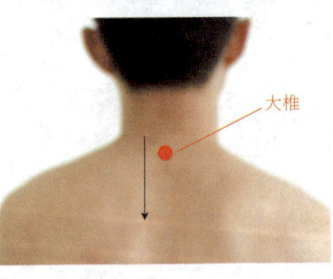

图52 大椎
Fig.52 Dazhui (GV 14)

刮，逐渐加重。

【注意事项】

1. 治疗时注意施术处的通风。

2. 治疗后嘱患者多喝水或口服补充生理盐水至少300～500ml。

3. 可根据患者的病症表现配服十滴水、千金消暑片等。

4. 若持续高热不退、神志昏迷，应及时送医急诊。

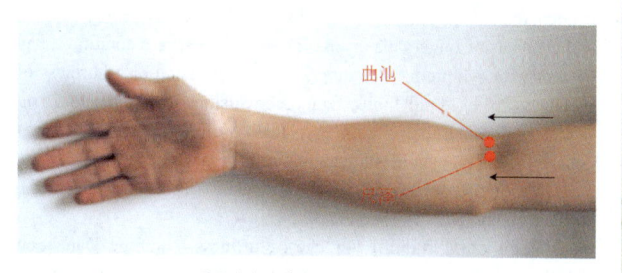

图53 曲池、尺泽
Fig.53 Quchi (LI 11) and Chize (LU 5)

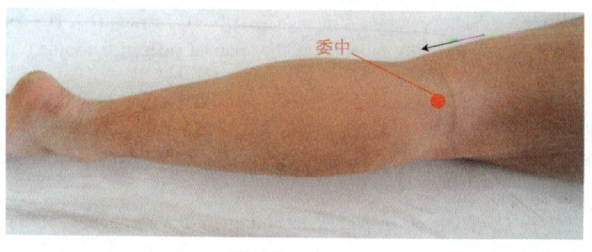

图54 委中
Fig.54 Weizhong (BL 40)

Chapter 9 Guasha Therapy for Internal Diseases

Section 1 Sunstroke

Sunstroke, also known as 'Fa Sha (eruption of Sha)', mostly occurs in summer. Those with a mild condition may present with sudden dizziness, headache, vexation, absence of sweating, nausea, and cyanosis of fingernails or lips. Those with a severe condition may present with symptoms including strong fever, agitation, shortness of breath, sweating, cold limbs, coma, convulsion or hypotension, and severe abdominal pain. Left untreated, high-grade fever, loss of consciousness or even life-threatening conditions may occur.

[Major points] Dazhui (GV 14), Quchi (LI 11), Chize (LU 5), and Weizhong (BL 40). (See Fig.52-54)

[Point combination] For chest stuffiness, combine Danzhong (CV 17); for nausea, combine Neiguan (PC 6); for coma, combine Renzhong (GV 26); for abdominal pain, combine Zhongwan (CV 12); and for headache, combine Yintang (EX-HN 3), Taiyang (EX-HN 5), and Fengchi (GB 20). In addition, the bilateral sides of the spine can also be scraped.

[Operation]

1. Scrape the major points with heavy pressure, creating 3 lines including the intended point and its bilateral sides until red spots or petechia appear.

2. Combine other points according to the symptoms of the patients. For headache, the practitioner can pinch Yintang (EX-HN 3)

until Sha marks appear, then push from Yintang (EX-HN 3) to Taiyang (EX-HN 5), and finally scrape from Taiyang (EX-HN 5) to Fengchi (GB 20); in addition, pinch Renzhong (GV 26) with fingers pointed towards the root of nose, and combine cupping on Tianshu (ST 25).

3. The practitioner can also directly scrape the bilateral sides of the spine in a downward direction with gradually increasing force.

[Cautionary notes]

1. Maintain good ventilation during the treatment.

2. Ask the patient to drink plenty of water or take at least 300-500 ml of normal saline orally.

3. Advise the patient to take patented Chinese medicine such as shí dī shuǐ and qiān jīn xiāo shǔ piàn (these are two examples of summer-heat removing tablets, which literally translates into Ten Drops of Water and Tablets Worth a Thousand Gold).

4. Send the patient for emergency treatment in case of persistent high-grade fever or coma.

第二节 发热

发热是指体温超过正常水平状态（36.2～37.2℃）。中医将发热分为外感与内伤发热两大类。外感发热多见高热、发病急剧，伴有恶寒等表证。内伤发热多见低热、持续时间长，主要由各种原发病证引起，以治疗原发病证为主。这里主要介绍外感发热的刮痧治疗。

【主穴】风池、大椎、曲池、风门、外关。（图55～56）

【配穴】咽痛咳嗽配列缺、鱼际、尺泽。

【操作方法】

1. 先重刮主穴各2～3行，直至痧痕出现为度。
2. 再根据随症刮拭配穴，以痧痕出现为止。
3. 也可取颈部向下至第四腰椎处顺刮，同时刮肘部、曲池穴。

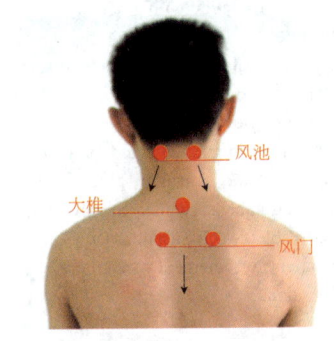

图55 大椎、风池、风门
Fig.55 Dazhui (GV 14), Fengchi (GB 20), and Fengmen (BL 12)

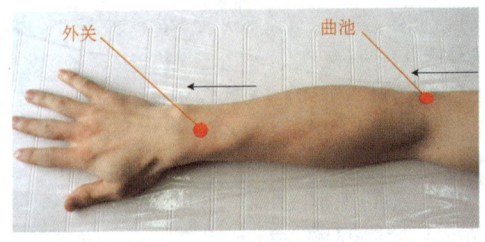

图56 外关、曲池
Fig.56 Waiguan (SJ 5) and Quchi (LI 11)

【注意事项】

1. 发热病症原因复杂，实施刮痧疗法前应注意判明原因。
2. 高热不退者，应及时送医就诊，采用综合治疗措施。
3. 刮痧前后应大量补充水分。结束时应覆被休息，避风寒。

Section 2 Fever

Fever refers to a condition in which the body temperature exceeds the normal range of 36.2-37.2℃. According to traditional Chinese medicine, fever can be caused by external contraction or internal injury. Those with external contraction usually present with symptoms of an exterior syndrome such as high grade fever, sudden onset, and aversion to cold. Those with internal injury usually present with persistent low-grade fever due to a variety of possible primary diseases. Here, Guasha therapy is mainly used for fever due to external contraction.

[Major points] Fengchi (GB 20), Dazhui (GV 14), Quchi (LI 11), Fengmen (BL 12), and Waiguan (SJ 5). (See Fig.55-56)

[Point combination] For sore throat and cough, combine with Lieque (LU 7), Yuji (LU 10), and Chize (LU 5).

[Operation]

1. Scrape the major points with heavy pressure, 2-3 lines for each point until red spots or petechia appear.

2. Combine other points on the basis of specific symptoms until Sha marks appear.

3. The practitioner can also scrape from the cervical area to L4, and scrape Quchi (LI 11) and the elbow area.

[Cautionary notes]

1. Since fever can be caused by complicated factors, the practitioner should be clear about the specific reason before commencing Guasha therapy.

2. Those with a persistent high-grade fever need to go to hospital for comprehensive measures.

3. Ask the patient to supplement water before and after Guasha, keep warm and take rest to avoid wind-cold after Guasha is complete.

第三节　感冒

感冒是以外感风邪为主的一种临床常见疾病。以恶寒发热、头痛鼻塞、喷嚏流涕、全身酸痛等症候为其特征。四季均可发病，以季节交替之际，气候变化骤然时多见，尤其是身体虚弱、老年、小儿易感。

【主穴】大椎、风池、风府、合谷、肺俞。（图57～59）

【配穴】头痛配印堂；头痛昏沉配百会；鼻塞配迎香；热甚配十宣。

【操作方法】

1. 先重刮，上从大椎下至肺俞、内从脊柱外至肩胛骨内侧缘区间，自上而下、自内而外刮拭3行。再刮其他主穴。

2. 根据病症轻重加刮配穴。如印堂撮至痧痕出现，太阳刮拭至耳前区间；百会穴向四周呈放射状刮拭；迎香、合谷点揉至皮肤微红为止；十宣选2～3点用消毒针点刺放血少许。

3. 也可取生姜、葱白各10g，切碎和匀布包，蘸热酒先刮前额、太阳穴，然后刮背部脊柱两侧，或配刮肘窝、腘窝。如有呕恶者加刮胸部。

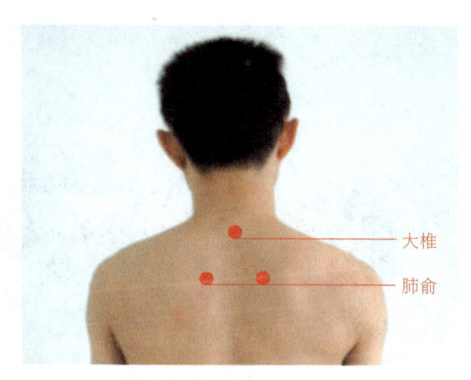

第九章　内科病症的刮痧疗法应用
Chapter 9　Guasha Therapy for Internal Diseases

图 57 大椎、肺俞
Fig.57 Dazhui (GV 14) and Feishu (BL 13)

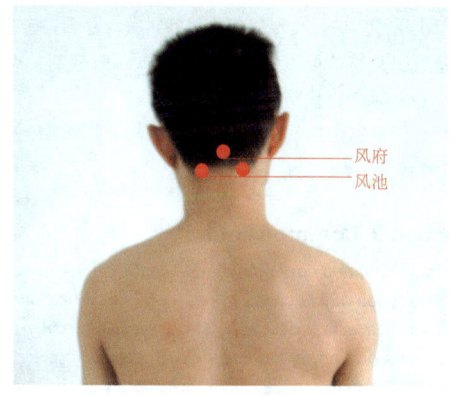

图 58 风府、风池
Fig.58 Fengfu (GV 16) and Fengchi (GB 20)

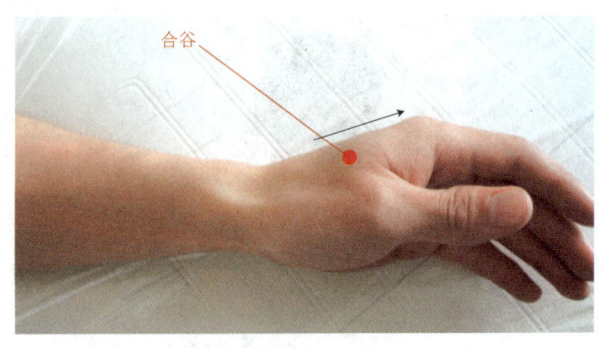

图 59 合谷
Fig.59 Hegu (LI 4)

【注意事项】

1. 每次治疗后应覆被保温避免风寒再袭。并嘱患者多饮水。

2. 感冒流行季节可服用板蓝根冲剂或每日轻刮、点揉足三里1次，连续3天予以预防。

3. 注意保持室内空气清新。季节交替，应加强身体锻炼，及时添减衣被。

Section 3 Common cold

Common cold is a common clinical condition mainly caused by external contraction of pathogenic wind. It is characterized by aversion to cold, fever, headache, nasal congestion, sneezing, runny nose, and general soreness or pain. It can occur in all seasons, especially at the change of season or sudden changes in weather. It easily attacks those with a weak constitution, the elderly, or children.

[Major points] Dazhui (GV 14), Fengchi (GB 20), Fengfu (GV 16), Hegu (LI 4), and Feishu (BL 13). (See Fig.57-59)

[Point combination] For headache, combine Yintang (EX-HN 3); for headache with dizziness, combine Baihui (GV 20); for nasal congestion, combine Yingxiang (LI 20); and for severe heat, combine Shixuan (EX-UE 11).

[Operation]

1. Scrape from Dazhui (GV 14) to Feishu (BL 13) and from the lateral aspect of the spine to medial border of the scapula with heavy pressure, 3 lines for each area, and then scrape other major points.

2. Combine other points according to specific symptoms. For example, pinch Yintang (EX-HN 3) until Sha marks appear; scrape from Taiyang (EX-HN 5) to the preauricular region; scrape from Baihui (GV 20) toward different directions; knead Yingxiang (LI 20) and Hegu (LI 4) until the local skin turns red; and apply blood-letting therapy (2-3 drops) to Shixuan (EX-UE 11).

3. The practitioner may also adopt 10g of fresh ginger and fistular onion stalk respectively, grind into a powder and wrap into a piece of cloth, dip the cloth into warm liquor and then scrape the forehead, Taiyang (EX-HN 5), bilateral sides of the spine or cubital fossa and popliteal fossa. For nausea and vomiting, scrape the chest area as well.

[Cautionary notes]

1. Keep warm after each treatment to avoid re-attack of wind cold and tell the patients to drink plenty of water.

2. In Flu season, take bǎn lán gēn (*Radix Isatidis*) granules, or scrape or knead Zusanli (ST 36) with mild force every day for three days to prevent cold.

3. Keep the air in the rooms at home fresh, exercise more at the

change of the season, and take care in sudden weather changes.

第四节　咳嗽

中医学认为咳嗽的病因有外感和内伤之分。外感咳嗽发病较急，病程短，常兼表证。若调治失当，可转为慢性咳嗽。内伤咳嗽病程较长，兼见胸脘痞闷、食少倦怠、胸胁引痛、面红舌赤等症。内伤咳嗽迁延失治，可并发喘息，称为"咳喘"。

【主穴】天突、膻中、尺泽、鱼际、肺俞。（图60～62）

【配穴】外感咳嗽配风池；内伤咳嗽配中府、脾俞、肾俞；胸闷配内关；痰多配足三里、丰隆；干咳配膏肓俞、三阴交。

【操作方法】

1. 先刮天突至膻中穴区间，再刮尺泽、鱼际、肺俞穴，至痧痕出现为止。

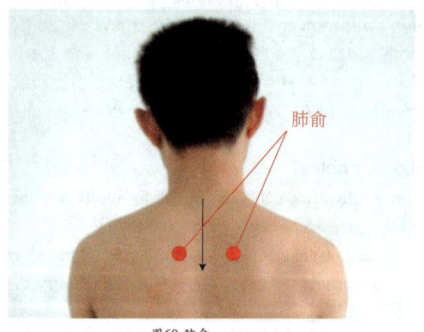

图60 *肺俞*
Fig.60 Feishu (BL 13)

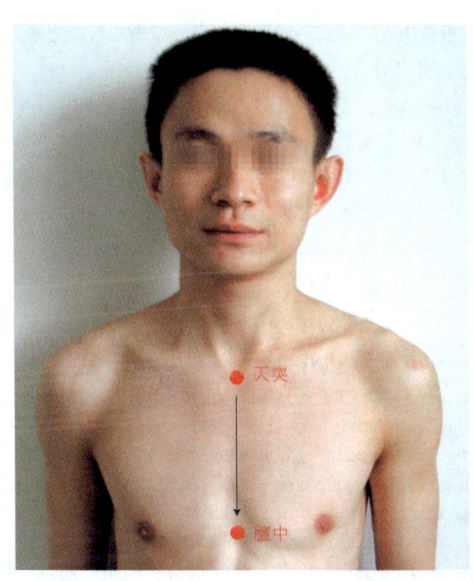

第九章　内科病症的刮痧疗法应用
Chapter 9　Guasha Therapy for Internal Diseases

图61 天突、膻中
Fig.61 Tiantu (CV 22) and Danzhong (CV 17)

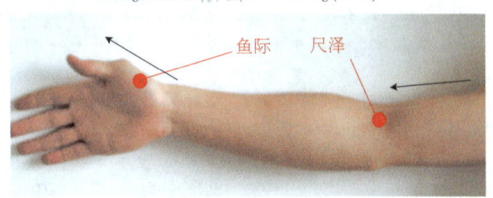

图62 鱼际、尺泽
Fig.62 Yuji (LU 10) and Chize (LU 5)

2. 根据出现的病症不同再刮配穴，以出现痧痕为度。

【注意事项】

1. 外感咳嗽、痰多者手法宜重，内伤气阴两虚，干咳气短者手法宜轻。

2. 对于咳嗽发作或初发咳嗽者有良好的效果，久病者应注意判明原因，并配合其他方法治疗。

3. 平时应注意锻炼身体，增强体质，预防感冒，戒烟戒酒。

Section 4 Cough

According to traditional Chinese medicine, cough can be caused by external contraction and an internal injury. Those with external contraction may present with sudden onset of a cough with a short duration and other symptoms of an exterior syndrome. Delayed or improper treatment may turn an acute cough into a chronic case. Those with an internal injury may present with a longer duration and symptoms such as fullness of chest or gastric region, a poor appetite, lassitude, radiating pain in chest and hypochondriac region, a red face and red tongue. Delayed or improper treatment may cause internal type cough to develop into panting, which is referred to as cough with dyspnea.

[Major points] Tiantu (CV 22), Danzhong (CV 17), Chize (LU 5), Yuji (LU 10), and Feishu (BL 13). (See Fig.60-62).

[Point combination] For cough due to external contraction, combine Fengchi (GB 20); for cough due to an internal injury, combine Zhongfu (LU 1), Pishu (BL 20), and Shenshu (BL 23); for stuffy chest, combine Neiguan (PC 6), for profuse phlegm, combine Zusanli (ST 36) and Fenglong (ST 40); and for unproductive cough, combine Gaohuangshu (BL 43) and Sanyinjiao (SP 6).

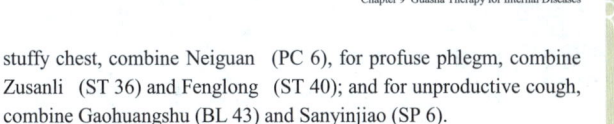

[Operation]

1. Scrape from Tiantu (CV 22) to Danzhong (CV 17), and then scrape Chize (LU 5), Yuji (LU 10), and Feishu (BL 13) until red spots or petechia appear.

2. Combine other points according to specific symptoms and scrape until Sha marks appear.

[Cautionary notes]

1. Use heavy stimulation for those with externally-contracted cough with profuse phlegm; and use mild stimulation for those with an unproductive cough with shortness of breath due to deficiency of qi and yin.

2. Guasha therapy works well in a coughing fit or at the early stages of a cough. For chronic cough, the practitioner should be clear about the true cause and combine with other therapies.

3. Do physical exercise to strengthen the body's constitution and prevent common cold, and cease smoking cigarettes or drinking alcohol.

第五节 哮喘

哮喘是一种反复发作性疾患。哮指喉中有痰鸣音，喘指呼吸困难而急促，两者常相兼而见。四季可发，以寒冷季节或气候骤变时发病较多。临床上分急性发作期和慢性缓解期。急性期可突然发作，多有喷嚏咽痒、胸闷气短等先兆症状，继而呼吸急促、气粗喘促、喉中哮鸣，甚者张口抬肩、不能平卧、口唇青紫、汗出肢冷等危重症候。

【主穴】发作期：大椎、肺俞、定喘、天突、膻中、中府、尺泽、鱼际。

缓解期：定喘、膏肓俞、脾俞、肾俞、中府、足三里、经渠。（图63～67）

【配穴】胸闷配内关；痰多配丰隆、足三里。

【操作方法】

1. 发作期：力度由轻至重，刮拭大椎和两侧定喘至肺俞，再刮天突至膻中、中府至前胸、尺泽至鱼际，由轻至重，至痧痕出现为度。

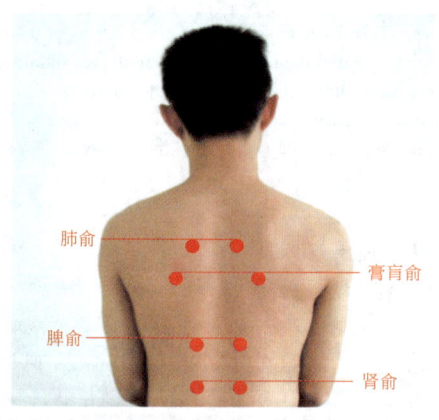

图63 肺俞、膏肓俞、脾俞、肾俞
Fig.63 Feishu (BL 13), Gaohuangshu (BL 43), Pishu (BL 20) and Shenshu (BL 23)

2. 缓解期：先轻刮定喘至膏肓俞区间，再刮两侧脾俞至肾俞区间，经渠至太渊，轻刮中府、足三里。以上均刮至皮肤出现痧痕为止。

3. 根据随症不同刮拭配穴。

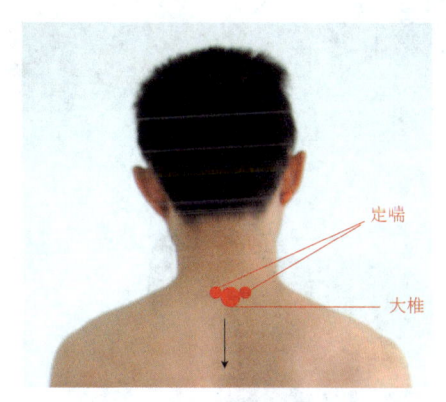

图64 定喘、大椎
Fig.64 Dingchuan (EX-B 1) and Dazhui (GV 14)

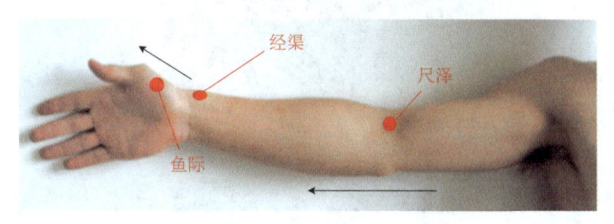

图65 鱼际、经渠、尺泽
Fig.65 Yuji (LU 10), Jingqu (LU 8), and Chize (LU 5)

下篇　刮痧疗法的实践应用
Part B Guasha Therapy in Practice

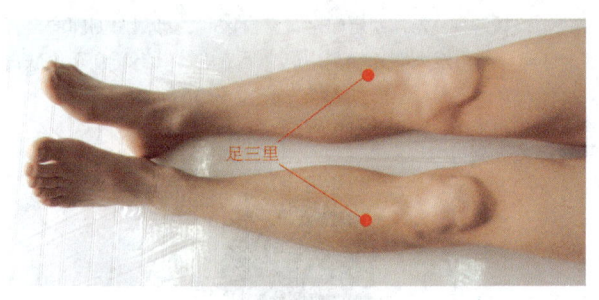

图66 足三里
Fig.66 Zusanli (ST 36)

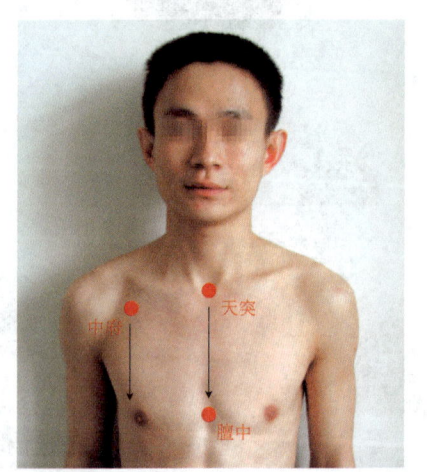

图67 中府、天突、膻中
Fig.67 Zhongfu (LU 1), Tiantu (CV 22), and Danzhong (CV 17)

【注意事项】

1. 发作严重或哮喘持续状态应配合其他药物治疗。

2. 缓解期应坚持治疗以巩固疗效,并适当加强体育锻炼以增强抗病能力,避免感冒。

3. 平日饮食宜清淡,注意避免接触致敏原和进食过敏食物。

4. 注意保暖防寒,戒烟酒,节性欲。

Section 5 Asthma

Asthma is a disorder characterized by recurrent attacks. Asthma is known in Chinese as xiào chuǎn. The first word refers to a wheezing sound and the second word refers to a rapid or difficult breathing. Asthma may occur in all seasons, especially in cold weather or upon sudden changes of weather. Clinically, two stages are seen; the acute attack stage and the chronic remission stage. Those with an acute attack may present with precursory symptoms such as sudden onset, sneezing, scratchy throat, chest stuffiness, and shortness of breath, followed by life-threatening symptoms including rapid breathing, panting with a wheezing sound, or even mouth breathing with raised shoulders, inability to lie flat, cyanosis of the lips, sweating, and cold limbs.

[Major points]

Acute stage: Dazhui (GV 14), Feishu (BL 13), Dingchuan (EX-B 1), Tiantu (CV 22), Danzhong (CV 17), Zhongfu (LU 1), Chize (LU 5), and Yuji (LU 10).

Remission stage: Dingchuan (EX-B 1), Gaohuangshu (BL 43), Pishu (BL 20), Shenshu (BL 23), Zhongfu (LU 1), Zusanli (ST 36), and Jingqu(LU 8). (See Fig.63-67)

[Point combination] For chest stuffiness, combine Neiguan (PC 6); and for profuse phlegm, combine Zusanli (ST 36) and Fenglong (ST 40).

[Operation]

1. Acute stage: Scrape from Dazhui (GV 14) and bilaterally from Dingchuan (EX-B 1) to Feishu (BL 13) with gradually increasing force, then scrape from Tiantu (CV 22) to Danzhong (CV 17), from Zhongfu (LU 1) to the prothorax, and from Chize (LU 5) to Yuji (LU 10) until Sha marks appear.

2. Remission stage: Scrape the area from Dingchuan (EX-B 1) to Gaohuangshu (BL 43) with mild force, then scrape bilaterally from Pishu (BL 20) to Shenshu (BL 23), from Jingqu (LU 8) to Taiyuan (LU 9), and finally scrape Zhongfu (LU 1) and Zusanli (ST 36) with mild force until Sha marks appear.

3. Scrape other points depending on specific symptoms.

[Cautionary notes]

1. Consider other medications in a severe attack or for persistent asthma.

2. Continue treatment in the remission stage to facilitate the therapeutic effect, and do more physical exercise to avoid common cold.

3. Eat bland food on a daily basis and stay away from sensitinogen or food that may cause an allergic reaction.

4. Keep warm, cease smoking cigarettes or drinking alcohol, and avoid sexual indulgence.

第六节 头痛

头痛是临床上常见的自觉症状。单独出现或见于其他急慢性疾病中。中医学认为"头为诸阳之会"，"脑为髓海"。无论外感风寒湿；或情志内伤，喜怒过度；或脏腑功能失调，肝肾不足等，均可引起头痛发作。表现为整个头部疼痛或前头、后枕、巅顶或偏侧的头痛。外感的头痛，多痛势骤起，痛剧无休，伴有表证；内伤头痛，多有反复，乍痛乍止或连绵不绝，伴有气滞血瘀或肝肾不足或肝阳上亢等里证。

【主穴】前头痛：印堂、合谷、神庭。

侧头痛：太阳、风池、率谷、阳辅。

巅顶痛：百会、太冲。

后枕痛：风府、天柱、昆仑。

全头痛：风池、大椎、合谷、太冲。（图52、58、59、68～72）

【配穴】外感头痛配列缺；内伤头痛配肝俞、肾俞、内关、三阴交、足三里。

【操作方法】

1. 根据头痛部位的不同先刮主穴，直至痧痕出现。

2. 再根据头痛的病症表现，分别刮拭所选配穴，以痧痕出现为度。

3. 有疼痛固定点的，用点揉法，每穴3～5分钟。

4. 天柱、印堂可用撮痧法。

【注意事项】

1. 对于初期或症状轻微的有明显的疗效。

2. 亦可预防头痛、消除疲劳。

3. 引起头痛的原因复杂，临床施用前应判明病因，特别是

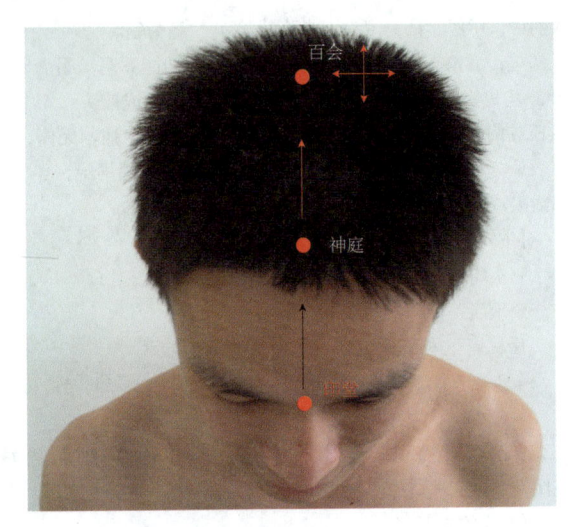

图68 百会、神庭、印堂
Fig.68 Baihui (GV 20), Shenting (GV 24), and Yintang (EX–HN 3)

颅脑器质性疾病引起的头痛，应及时治疗原发病。

Section 6 Headache

Headache is a common subjective symptom. It can occur alone or as a result of other acute or chronic disorders. Traditional Chinese medicine asserts that the 'head is the gathering place of all yang', and the 'brain is the sea of marrow'. According to the TCM theory, headache can be caused by the following factors: external contraction of wind, cold and dampness; internal injury due to excessive joy or

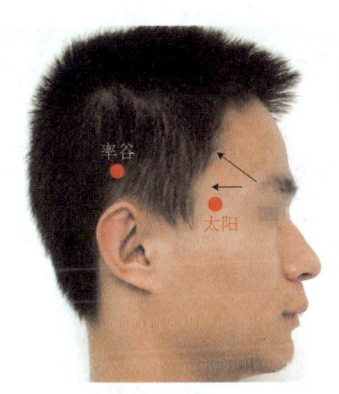

第九章　内科病症的刮痧疗法应用
Chapter 9 Guasha Therapy for Internal Diseases

图 69 率谷、太阳
Fig.69 Shuaigu (GB 8), and Taiyang (EX-HN 5)

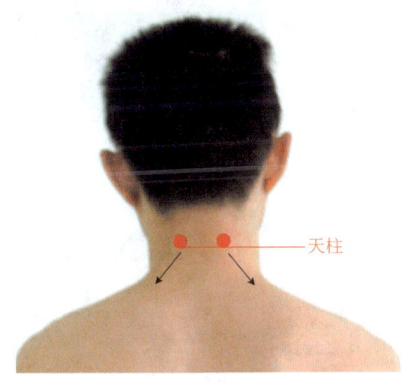

图 70 天柱
Fig.70 Tianzhu (BL 10)

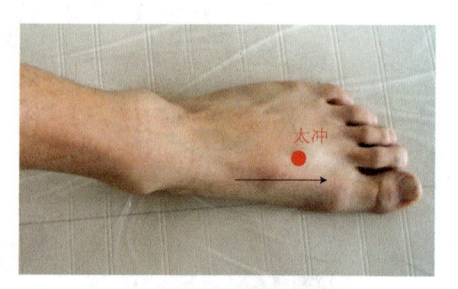

图71 太冲
Fig.71 Taichong (LR 3)

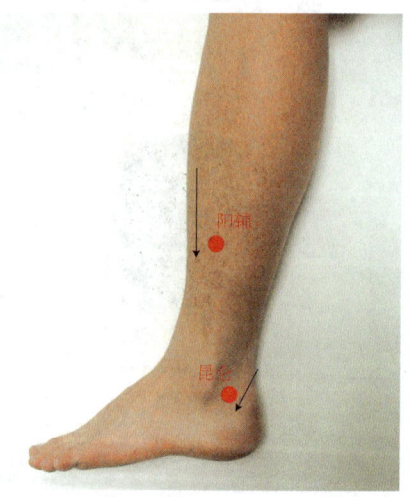

图72 阳辅、昆仑
Fig.72 Yangfu (GB 38) and Kunlun (BL 60)

anger; dysfunction of the zang-fu organs such as deficiency of the liver and kidney. Headache can occur in the whole head, frontal, occipital, on the vertex or lateral sides. Those with external contraction may present with sudden, severe headache with symptoms of an exterior syndrome. Those with an internal injury may present with recurrent, intermittent or lingering headache, along with symptoms of an interior syndrome including qi and blood stagnation, deficiency of the liver and kidney, or hyperactivity of liver-yang.

[Major points]

Frontal headache: Yintang (EX-HN 3), Hegu (LI 4), and Shenting (GV 24).

Migraine: Taiyang (EX-HN 5), Fengchi (GB 20), Shuaigu (GB 8), and Yangfu (GB 38).

Parietal headache: Baihui (GV 20) and Taichong (LR 3).

Occipital headache: Fengfu (GV 16), Tianzhu (BL 10), and Kunlun (BL 60).

General headache: Fengchi (GB 20), Dazhui (GV 14), Hegu (LI 4), and Taichong (LR 3). (See Fig.52, 58, 59, 68-72)

[Point combination] For headache due to external contraction, combine Lieque (LU 7); for headache due to internal injury, combine Ganshu (BL 18), Shenshu (BL 23), Neiguan (PC 6), Sanyinjiao (SP 6), and Zusanli (ST 36).

[Operation]

1. Scrape the major points according to location of the headache until Sha marks appear.

2. Combine other points depending on specific symptoms until Sha marks appear.

3. Apply kneading manipulation for fixed pain, 3-5 minutes on each point.

4. Apply the twisting method for Tianzhu (BL 10) and Yintang (EX-HN 3).

[Cautionary notes]

1. Guasha works effectively for early-stage or mild headache.
2. Guasha can also prevent headache and relieve fatigue.
3. Since headache can be caused by complicated factors, the practitioner should be clear about the specific reason and treat the primary disease as early as possible. This is especially true of organic diseases of the cranium.

第七节 失眠

失眠专指经常不易入睡，或睡眠时间短，或睡眠不深，甚者彻夜不眠的病症。排除因一时情绪紧张或环境不宁、卧榻不适等因素或因发热、咳喘、疼痛等疾病引起的失眠。

【主穴】背部脊柱两旁、印堂、百会、神门、三阴交。（图73～76)

【配穴】气血不足配足三里、心俞、脾俞；阴虚火旺配肾俞、大陵；痰湿重配中脘、丰隆、足三里；肝火上扰配太冲、风池、期门。

【操作方法】

1. 先刮拭脊柱两旁的背俞穴，重刮心俞、神堂之间，以皮肤潮红即可。

2. 呈星状放射刮拭，从百会刮向四周，至局部温热感。

3. 印堂向上发根处刮拭、神门向上、三阴交向下刮拭至内踝后侧，以皮肤潮红为度。

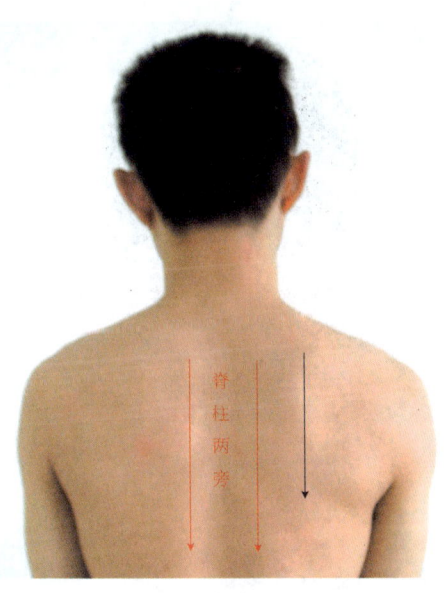

第九章　内科病症的刮痧疗法应用
Chapter 9 Guasha Therapy for Internal Diseases

图 73 脊柱两旁
Fig.73 Bilateral sides of the spine

4. 根据病症刮拭配穴。

【注意事项】

1. 加强身体锻炼，合理安排饮食起居。

2. 注意消除引起失眠的因素，适当予以心理指导，有助于病情的康复。

下篇 刮痧疗法的实践应用
Part B Guasha Therapy in Practice

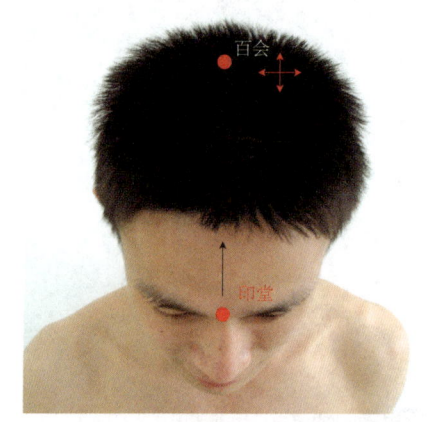

图 74 百会、印堂
Fig.74 Baihui (GV 20) and Yintang (EX-HN 3)

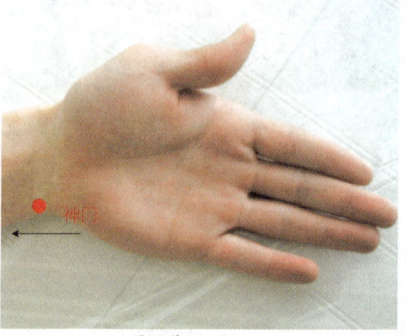

图 75 神门
Fig.75 Shenmen (HT 7)

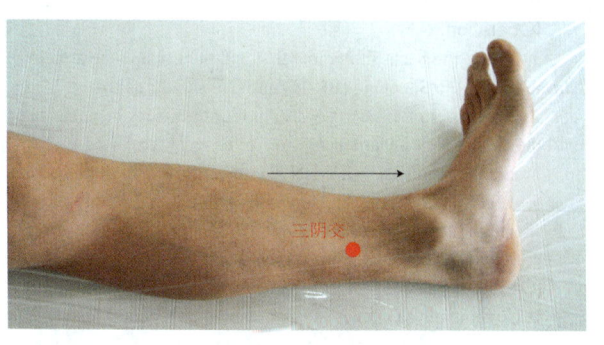

图 76 三阴交
Fig.76 Sanyinjiao (SP 6)

Section 7 Insomnia

Insomnia refers to disorders including difficulty falling asleep, short hours of sleep, easily-disturbed sleep, or even sleeplessness throughout the night. Factors such as emotional nervousness, a noisy environment, an uncomfortable bed, fever, cough, or pain should be excluded.

[Major points] Bilateral sides along the spine, Yintang (EX-HN 3), Baihui (GV 20), Shenmen (HT 7), and Sanyinjiao (SP 6). (See Fig. 73-76)

[Point combination] For deficiency of qi and blood, combine Zusanli (ST 36), Xinshu (BL 15), and Pishu (BL 20); for hyperactivity of fire due to yin deficiency, combine Shenshu (BL 23) and Daling (PC 7); for phlegm-dampness, combine Zhongwan (CV 12), Fenglong (ST 40), and Zusanli (ST 36); and for upwards counterflow of liver-fire, combine Taichong (LR 3), Fengchi (GB 20), and Qimen (LR 14).

[Operation]

1. Scrape the back-Shu points first and then scrape the area from Xinshu (BL 15) to Shentang (BL 44) until the skin turns red.

2. Scrape from Baihui (GV 20) in four directions in a star shape until the patient feels a warm sensation in the local area.

3. Scrape Yintang (EX-HN 3) towards the hairline, scrape Shenmen (HT 7) upwards, and scrape Sanyinjiao (SP 6) downwards, to the posterior aspect of the medial malleolus, until the skin turns red.

4. Scrape other points according to specific symptoms.

[Cautionary notes]

1. Do more physical exercise and maintain a regular lifestyle.

2. Avoid factors that may cause insomnia and appropriate psychological counseling may help.

第八节 胁痛

胁痛是以一侧或两侧胁肋部疼痛为主要表现的病证。临床多分为实证和虚证两类。前者与情绪、饮食肥甘、跌仆损伤有关；后者多由前者经久不愈或年高体弱多见。

【主穴】脊柱两旁的背俞穴、日月、期门、支沟、阳陵泉。（图73、77~79）

【配穴】肝气郁结配太冲；气滞血瘀配三阴交；肝胆湿热配外关、侠溪；气血不足配肝俞、肾俞、脾俞、三阴交。

【操作方法】

1. 先刮拭脊柱两旁的背俞穴，重刮膈俞、肝俞、胆俞之间，以皮肤潮红即可。

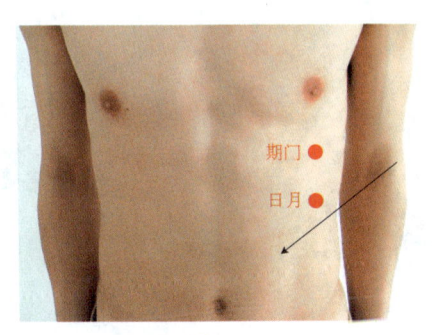

第九章　内科病症的刮痧疗法应用
Chapter 9 Guasha Therapy for Internal Diseases

图 77 期门、日月
Fig.77 Qimen (LR 14) and Riyue (GB 24)

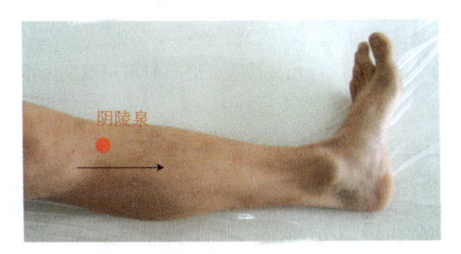

图 78 阴陵泉
Fig.78 Yinlingquan (SP 9)

2. 呈扇形状放射刮拭，从日月、期门刮向胁下，至局部温热感。

3. 支沟、阳陵泉分别向下刮拭至腕关节和外踝，以皮肤潮红为度。

4. 根据病症刮拭配穴。

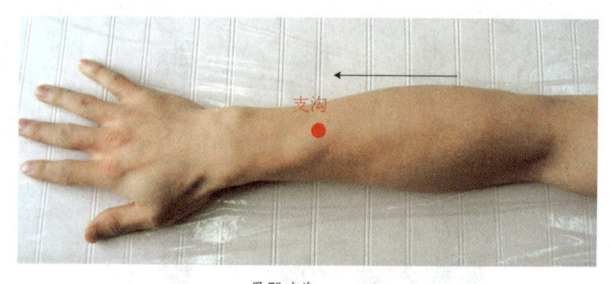

图 79 支沟
Fig.79 Zhigou (SJ 6)

【注意事项】

1. 调整饮食起居，保持心情愉悦。
2. 治疗同时须进行相关检查，必要时可采取病因治疗。

Section 8 Hypochondriac pain

Hypochondriac pain is mainly characterized by unilateral or bilateral pain in the hypochondriac region. According to traditional Chinese medicine, it can be caused by both excessive and deficient syndrome. The excessive patterns are associated with factors such as emotions, an improper diet, or traumatic injuries, whereas deficient patterns are usually caused by a long duration of an excessive pattern and the aging process.

[Major points] Back-shu points, Riyue (GB 24), Qimen (LR 14), Zhigou (SJ 6), and Yanglingquan (GB 34). (See Fig.73, 77-79)

[Point combination] For liver-qi stagnation, combine Taichong (LR 3); for qi stagnation and blood stasis, combine Sanyinjiao (SP 6);

for damp-heat in the liver and gallbladder, combine Waiguan (SJ 5) and Xiaxi (GB 43); and for deficiency of qi and blood, combine Ganshu (BL 18), Shenshu (BL 23), Pishu (BL 20), and Sanyinjiao (SP 6).

[Operation]

1. Scrape the back-Shu point first with especially with heavy force on the area from Geshu (BL 17), to Ganshu (BL 18) and Danshu (BL 19) until the skin turns red.

2. Scrape Riyue (GB 24) and Qimen (LR 14) downwards to the hypochondriac region in a fan shape until the patient feels a warm sensation in the local area.

3. Scrape Zhigou (SJ 6) and Yanglingquan (GB 34) down to wrist joint and external malleolus until the skin turns red.

4. Combine other points according to specific symptoms.

[Cautionary notes]

1. Regulate the lifestyle and maintain a peaceful mind.

2. Do relevant examinations during the treatment and treat the primary cause if necessary.

第九节 呕吐

呕吐是由多种原因引起胃失和降、气逆于上，表现以胃内容物突然上逆吐出的一种临床症状。可见于多种疾病中。外感风寒暑湿，或过食生冷油腻，痰湿困于脾胃，或恼怒伤肝，气逆犯脾，或脾胃气虚，水谷不化等为常见致病因素。

【主穴】足三里、膻中、中脘、内关。（图66、80、81）

【配穴】呕吐热臭配合谷、内庭；呕吐清水或稀涎配上脘、公孙；呕吐痰涎配足三里、丰隆；呕吐宿食配璇玑、腹通谷、下

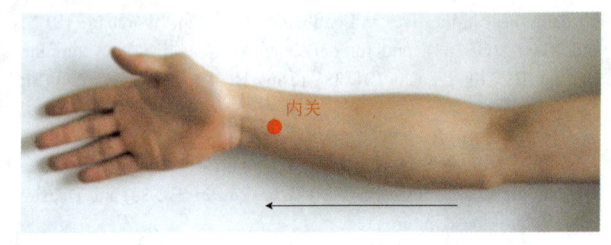

图 80 内关
Fig.80 Neiguan (PC 6)

脘；呕吐泛酸、精神抑郁配阳陵泉、太冲、期门；呕吐时作、脾胃虚弱配肾俞、脾俞、胃俞、章门。

【操作方法】

1. 先点揉内关、公孙，至穴区热、胀，皮肤泛红为度。

2. 从中脘向脐、膻中向下、足三里向踝部刮拭至痧痕出现。

3. 根据病情刮拭配穴。

【注意事项】

1. 饮食宜清淡、易消化。避免进食生冷、油腻、煎炸、辛辣食物。

2. 呕吐严重者应送医院进行综合治疗，及时补液以纠正电解质紊乱。

3. 注意探明呕吐的原因，注意对原发病的治疗。对于妊娠呕吐可参照上述治疗，但应注意穴位的选取，且操作力度应轻柔。

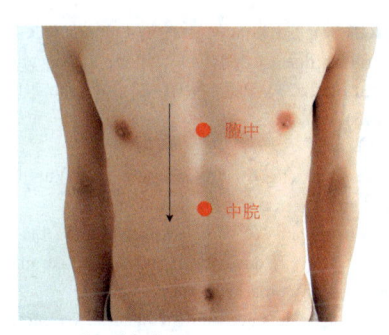

图 81 膻中 中脘
Fig.81 Danzhong (CV 17) and Zhongwan (CV 12)

Section 9 Vomiting

Vomiting is a clinical symptom caused by adverse up-flow of stomach-qi due to a variety of reasons. It can occur as a result of many conditions. The common etiological factors include external contraction of wind, cold, summer-heat, and dampness, ingestion of raw, cold, and oily food, dam phlegm retention in the spleen and stomach, liver-qi attacking the spleen, or poor digestion due to qi deficiency of the spleen and stomach

[Major points] Zusanli (ST 36), Danzhong (CV 17), Zhongwan (CV 12), and Neiguan (PC 6). (See Fig.66, 80, 81)

[Point combination] For vomiting with foul breath, combine Hegu (LI 4) and Neiting (ST 44); for hydroptysis or thin drool, combine Shangwan (CV 13) and Gongsun (SP 4); for vomiting with phlegm, combine Zusanli (ST 36) and Fenglong (ST 40); for vomiting of undigested food, combine Xuanji (CV 21), Futonggu (KI 20), and Xiawan (CV 10); for acid reflux and mental depression, combine

Yanglingquan (GB 34), Taichong (LR 3), and Qimen (LR 14); and for intermittent vomiting due to deficiency of the spleen and stomach, combine Shenshu (BL 23), Pishu (BL 20), Weishu (BL 21) and Zhangmen (LR 13).

[Operation]

1. Knead Neiguan (PC 6) and Gongsun (SP 4) until the patient feels warm and distended in the local area.

2. Scrape Zhongwan (CV 12) downwards to the umbilicus, scrape Danzhong (CV 17) downward, and scrape Zusanli (ST 36) towards the ankle until Sha marks appear.

3. Combine other points according to specific symptoms.

[Cautionary notes]

1. Eat bland and easy-to-digest food; and stay away from raw, cold, oily, fried or spicy food.

2. Those with severe vomiting need comprehensive therapy and immediate fluid infusion to correct electrolyte disturbances.

3. The practitioner should be clear about the true cause of vomiting. However, for vomiting in pregnancy, take care in selecting points and use gentle force.

第十节 呃逆

呃逆，又称"哕逆"。是指胃气上逆动膈，气逆上冲，喉间呃呃连声，声短而频，不能自止为主要表现的病证。常受情绪、饮食影响，临床以偶然发生者居多，为时短暂，多可自愈，有的则屡屡发生，持续时间较长，常伴有胸膈痞闷，脘中不适，情绪不安等。现在医学中的单纯性膈肌痉挛即属呃逆。

【主穴】膈俞、膈关、内关、翳风、日月、期门、水沟、膻

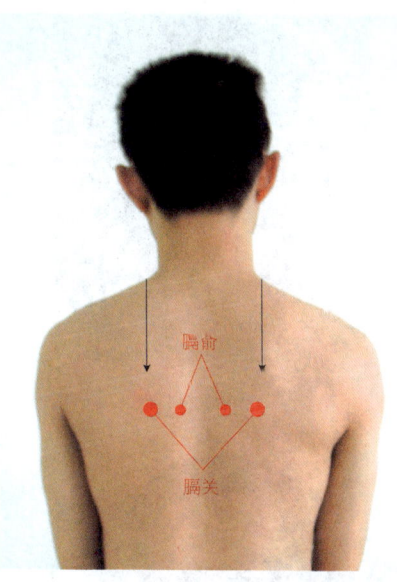

第九章　内科病症的刮痧疗法应用
Chapter 9　Guasha Therapy for Internal Diseases

图 82 膈俞 膈关
Fig.82 Geshu (BL 17) and Geguan (BL 46)

中、天突。（图67、77、80、82～84）

【配穴】脾胃虚寒配中脘、足三里；胃阴不足配三阴交、内庭、太溪；气机郁滞配太冲、阳陵泉；病久体虚配脊柱两侧背俞穴、足三里、关元。

【操作方法】

1. 膈俞、膈关、内关分别点按至酸胀感，再刮拭至皮肤潮红

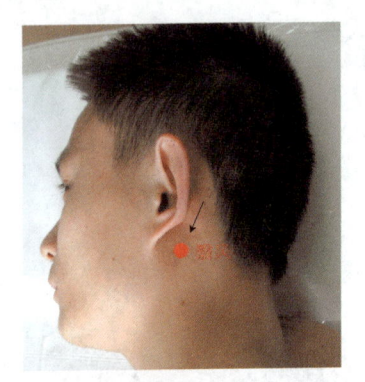

图 83 翳风
Fig.83 Yifeng (SJ 17)

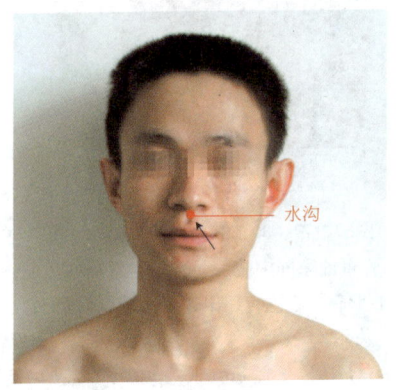

图 84 水沟
Fig.84 Shuigou (GV 26)

或瘀痕出现。

2. 翳风点按酸胀后向下颈项刮拭至皮肤潮红。

3. 日月、期门呈扇形向胁肋刮拭至皮肤潮红。

4. 水沟向鼻根部点按。

5. 膻中、天突向胸骨刮拭至皮肤潮红。

6. 随症刮拭配穴。

【注意事项】

1. 避免清冷饮食,调和情志。

2. 其他疾病如胃肠神经症、胃炎、胃扩张、胃癌、肝硬化晚期、脑血管病、尿毒症,以及胃、食管手术后等所引起的膈肌痉挛,则应以治疗原发病证为主。

Section 10 Hiccups

Hiccups, also known as non-productive vomiting, refer to short, constant, and involuntary retching due to the upwards flow of stomach qi. It is often related to the emotions and diet. Clinically it occurs accidentally and temporarily and can stop spontaneously. However, some people may experience frequent and persistent hiccups, along with symptoms such as chest stuffiness, gastric discomfort, and emotional disturbances. The simple diaphragmatic spasm in modern medicine is also ascribed to hiccups.

[Major points] Geshu (BL 17), Geguan (BL 46), Neiguan (PC 6), Yifeng (SJ 17), Riyue (GB 24), Qimen (LR 14), Shuigou (GV 26), Danzhong (CV 17), and Tiantu (CV 22) .(See Fig.67, 77, 80, 82-84)

[Point combination] For deficient cold in the spleen and stomach, combine Zhongwan (CV 12) and Zusanli (ST 36); for stomach-yin deficiency, combine Sanyinjiao (SP 6), Neiting (ST 44), and Taixi (KI 3); for qi stagnation, combine Taichong (LR 3) and Yanglingquan (GB 34); and for a weak constitution due to a chronic condition, combine back-Shu points, Zusanli (ST 36), and Guanyuan (CV 4)

[Operation]

1. Press Geshu (BL 17), Geguan (BL 46), and Neiguan (PC 6) until the patient feels soreness and distension and then scrape these points until the skin turns red or Sha marks appear.

2. Press Yifeng (SJ 17) until the patient feels soreness and distension and then scrape downwards to the nape until the skin turns red.

3. Scrape Riyue (GB 24) and Qimen (LR 14) in a fan shape toward hypochondriac region until the skin turns red.

4. Press Renzhong (GV 26) towards the root of the nose.

5. Scrape other points according to specific symptoms.

[Cautionary notes]

1. Avoid cold food and maintain a peaceful mind.

2. Treat primary disorders such as gastrointestinal neurosis, gastritis, gastrectasia, gastric cancer, late stage of liver cirrhosis, cerebrovascular disease, uremia, and diaphragmatic spasm due to stomach or esophagus operation.

第十一节　胃痛

胃痛是指以上腹胃脘部近心窝处出现反复发作性疼痛为主症的自觉证候，又称为"胃脘痛"。中医学认为，胃痛多因寒邪客于胃脘，或忧思恼怒，肝郁犯胃，或素体虚弱，又因饮食不慎，或思虑劳累等引起。

【主穴】梁丘、至阳、内关、足三里。（图80、85、86）

【配穴】寒邪客胃配脾俞、胃俞；饮食停滞配梁门、天枢、大肠俞；肝郁犯胃配期门、章门、太冲；中焦虚寒配脾俞、胃俞、中脘、肾俞、足三里、气海；胃痛日久，气滞血瘀配膈俞、三阴交、公孙。

【操作方法】

1. 至阳、梁丘、内关、足三里分别先点按至酸胀感，再刮拭至皮肤潮红或痧痕出现。

2. 根据病情辨证加刮配穴。

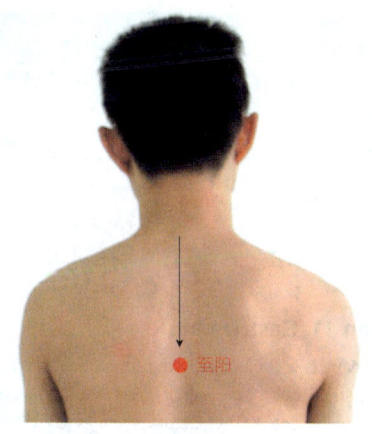

图85 至阳
Fig.85 Zhiyang (GV 9)

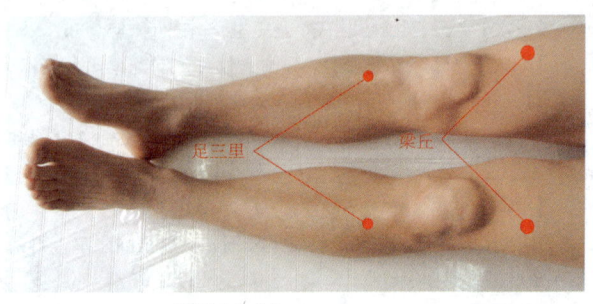

图86 足三里、梁丘
Fig.86 Zusanli (ST 36) and Liangqiu (ST 34)

【注意事项】

1. 注意探明胃痛的原因，注意与肝胆疾患或胰腺炎等的鉴别。

2. 对于溃疡出血、穿孔等重症，应及时送医院采取综合措施或手术治疗。

3. 注意饮食、起居、情志的调节。平日宜少食多餐，禁食生冷、辛辣、煎炸或过于油腻肥甘的食物。忌烟酒。

Section 11 Gastric pain

Gastric pain is a subjective symptom characterized by recurrent pain in epigastric area. Traditional Chinese medicine asserts that gastric pain can be caused by factors such as cold retention in the stomach, anxiety, liver-qi attacking the stomach, constitutional weakness plus improper diet or fatigue.

[Major points] Liangqiu (ST 34), Zhiyang (GV 9), Neiguan (PC 6), and Zusanli (ST 36) .(See Fig.80, 85, 86)

[Point combination] For cold retention in the stomach, combine Pishu (BL 20) and Weishu (BL 21); for food retention, combine Liangmen (ST 21), Tianshu (ST 25), and Dachangshu (BL 25); for liver-qi attacking the stomach, combine Qimen (LR 14), Zhangmen (LR 13), and Taichong (LR 3); for deficient cold in the middle jiao, combine Pishu (BL 20), Weishu (BL 21), Zhongwan (CV 12), Shenshu (BL 23), Zusanli (ST 36), and Qihai (CV 6); and for qi stagnation and blood stasis due to chronic gastric pain, combine Geshu (BL 17), Sanyinjiao (SP 6), and Gongsun (SP 4).

[Operation]

1. Knead points Zhiyang (GV 9), Liangqiu (ST 34), Neiguan (PC 6), and Zusanli (ST 36) until the patient feels soreness and distension and then scrape until the skin turns red or Sha marks appear.

2. Scrape other points according to specific symptoms.

[Cautionary notes]

1. Gastric pain should be differentiated from liver or gallbladder conditions or from pancreatitis before commencing Guasha therapy.

2. Those with life-threatening conditions such as ulcerative bleeding or perforation should be sent to hospital immediately for comprehensive therapy or surgery.

3. Regulate dietary habits and lifestyle, maintain a peaceful mind, eat more frequently but decrease the amount for each meal, stay away from raw, cold, spicy, fried or oily food, and cease smoking cigarettes or drinking alcohol.

第十二节 便秘

便秘是指大便涩滞、秘结不通,秘结时间超过2天以上,或虽有便意但排便困难的病证。多因阳盛之人又嗜食辛辣煎炸食物,或忧思恼怒、情志不畅,或病后、产后、年老体衰,气血两虚,阳气不足等因素所致。

【主穴】天枢、左腹结、大肠俞、上巨虚、支沟。(图79、87~89)

【配穴】热秘配合谷、内庭;肝郁气秘配太冲;气血不足配膈俞、脾俞;阳气不足配气海、关元、命门、肾俞;年老津亏配太溪。

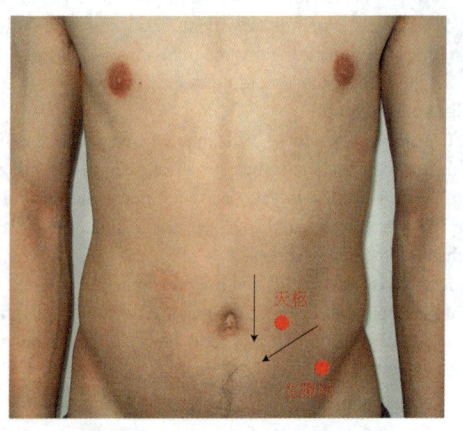

图87 天枢 左腹结
Fig.87 Tianshu (ST 25) and Fujie (SP 14) in the left side

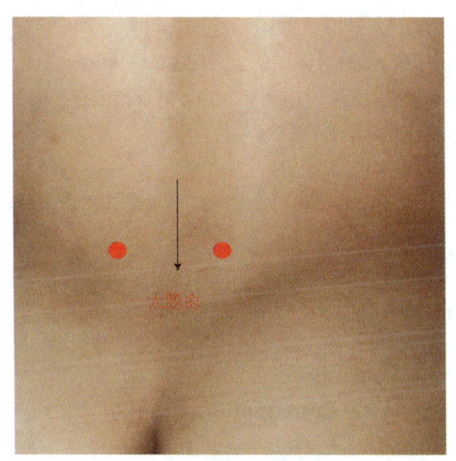

第九章　内科病症的刮痧疗法应用
Chapter 9　Guasha Therapy for Internal Diseases

图88 大肠俞
Fig.88 Dachangshu (BL 25)

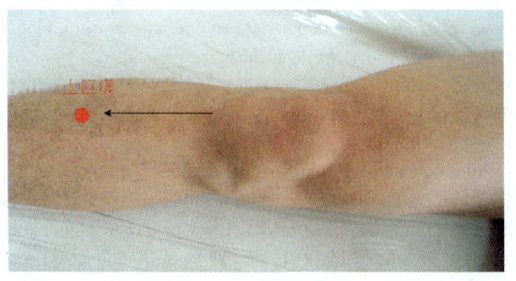

图89 上巨虚
Fig.89 Shangjuxu (ST 37)

【操作方法】

1. 左腹结向腹股沟方向，上巨虚、天枢穴向下，大肠俞向骶部，支沟穴向腕部方向刮拭，以皮肤潮红或至痧痕出现为止。

2. 根据病情辨证刮拭配穴。

【注意事项】

1. 注意饮食调节，平时多食蔬菜水果等富含水分和纤维食物。

2. 注意适当身体锻炼。

3. 注意养成按时排便的习惯。排便前后可自行进行脐周按摩，以局部热感为度。

Section 12 Constipation

Constipation refers to a condition of unsmooth defecation, not more than one bowel movement in more than 2 days, or difficult defecating. Traditional Chinese medicine asserts that constipation can be caused by factors such as excessive yang with a preference for spicy and fried food, emotional depression, and deficiency of qi, blood, and yang due to disease, childbirth, or the aging process.

[Major points] Tianshu (ST 25), Fujie (SP 14) in the left side, Dachangshu (BL 25), Shangjuxu (ST 37), and Zhigou (SJ 6). (See Fig. 79, 87-89)

[Point combination] For heat constipation, combine Hegu (LI 4) and Neiting (ST 44); for constipation due to liver-qi stagnation, combine Taichong (LR 3); for deficiency of qi and blood, combine Geshu (BL 17) and Pishu (BL 20); for yang-qi deficiency, combine Qihai (CV 6), Guanyuan (CV 4), Mingmen (GV 4), and Shenshu (BL

23); and for insufficiency of liquid due to aging process, combine Taixi (KI 3).

[Operation]

1. Scrape Fujie (SP 14) on the left side towards the groin, scrape Shangjuxu (ST 37) and Tianshu (ST 25) downwards, scrape Dachangshu (BL 25) towards the sacral region, and scrape Zhigou (SJ 6) towards the wrist until the skin turns red or Sha marks appear.

2. Scrape other points according to specific symptoms.

[Cautionary notes]

1. Regulate dietary habits and eat foods that are rich in water and fiber such as vegetables and fruits.

2. Do appropriate physical exercise.

3. Have regular defecation and massage peri-umbilical area before or after defecation until a local warm sensation appears.

第十三节 眩晕

眩晕是一种临床常见的自觉症状。眩指眼花，晕指头旋，常同时出现。轻者发作短暂，休息片刻即可缓解；重者如坐舟车，旋转不宁，站立困难，并伴有恶心呕吐、头痛头胀等症。中医学认为，情志失调又嗜食肥甘，风痰上扰清空或房事不节、过度劳作，髓海空虚，均可导致眩晕。

【主穴】百会、风府、风池、合谷、太冲。（图58、59、71、74）

【配穴】体虚者配膈俞、脾俞、足三里；烦躁易怒，肝阳上亢者配率谷、风池、风市、阳陵泉；舌苔厚浊，痰湿重者配阴陵泉、地机、足三里、丰隆；腰酸耳鸣，肝肾不足者配肾俞、志室、腰阳关、气海、关元。

【操作方法】

1. 百会穴向外呈星状放射刮拭,用力轻柔,以局部温热即可。

2. 风府、风池穴向下刮拭,至出现痧痕为止。

3. 合谷、太冲穴先点揉至酸胀感,再刮拭,以皮肤潮红为度。

4. 根据病症刮拭配穴,体虚肝肾不足应采用轻手法,至皮肤泛红为止。

【注意事项】

1. 头晕发作时,应安卧或安坐、闭目休息并做和缓均匀的呼吸,保持室内空气流通。

2. 可配合做眼球揉按或穴位指压,如印堂、太阳、合谷等辅助按摩方法,有助于提高疗效。

3. 应探明眩晕引发的原因,及时治疗原发病证,对于长期使用链霉素、卡那霉素等抗生素患者,治疗效果较差。

Section 13 Vertigo

Vertigo is a common subjective symptom. It is known in Chinese as xuàn yūn. The first word means dizziness or blurry vision, and the second word means a spinning head. Those with a mild condition may recover without treatment after some time. Those with a severe condition may feel like they are sitting in a boat and present with symptoms such as dystasia, nausea, vomiting, headache, and a distending sensation of the head. Traditional Chinese medicine assert that factors including emotional disturbance, excessive ingestion of sweet and fatty food, wind-phlegm disturbing the mind, sexual indulgence, fatigue, or brain deficiency may play a role in vertigo.

[Major points] Baihui (GV 20), Fengfu (GV 16), Fengchi (GB 20), Hegu (LI 4), and Taichong (LR 3). (See Fig.58, 59, 71, 74)

[Point combination] For a weak constitution, combine Geshu (BL 17), Pishu (BL 20) and Zusanli (ST 36); for irritability due to hyperactivity of liver-yang, combine Shuaigu (GB 8), Fengchi (GB 20), Fengshi (GB 31), and Yanglingquan (GB 34); for a thick and turbid tongue coating due to phlegm-dampness, combine Yinlingquan (SP 9), Diji (SP 8), Zusanli (ST 36), and Fenglong (ST 40); and for lumbar soreness and tinnitus due to deficiency of the liver and kidney, combine Shenshu (BL 23), Zhishi (BL 52), Yaoyangguan (GV 3), Qihai (CV 6), and Guanyuan (CV 4).

[Operation]

1. Scrape Baihui (GV 20) outwards in a star shape with a gentle force until the patients feel warm in the local area.

2. Scrape Fengfu (GV 16) and Fengchi (GB 21) downwards until Sha marks appear.

3. Knead Hegu (LI 4) and Taichong (LR 3) until the patient feels soreness and distension and scrape until the skin turns red.

4. Scrape other points according to specific symptoms and use mild stimulation for those with a weak constitution due to deficiency of the liver and kidney, until the skin turns red.

[Cautionary notes]

1. During an attack of dizziness, lie or sit down, close one's eyes, breathe evenly, and maintain good ventilation.

2. Massage the eyeball or apply finger pressure to points such as Yintang (EX-HN 3), Taiyang (EX-HN 5) and Hegu (LI 4).

3. Treat the possible primary cause for vertigo. Those with long-term use of streptomycin and kanamycin may not respond well to Guasha therapy.

第十四节 高血压

高血压是最常见的心血管疾病之一，以中老年人发病居多。其最主要的临床特点是动脉压增高，可表现收缩压或舒张压升高或两者均升高，即收缩压≥140mmHg，舒张压≥90mmHg。长期高血压可影响心、脑、肾等重要脏器的功能，甚至导致脏器功能衰竭而病残或死亡。中医学认为，本病多因年老体弱或忧思过度、饮食肥甘厚味食物、精神紧张或受强烈刺激等所致。

【主穴】夹脊穴、脊柱两侧背俞穴、风池、肩井、合谷、太冲。（图59、71、90~91）

【配穴】饮食肥甘厚味，体形肥胖，痰湿重者配百会、风府、足三里、丰隆；年老体虚，肝肾不足者配三阴交、太溪、涌泉；烦躁易怒，肝胆火旺者配头临泣、风池、风市、阳陵泉；效果不好者配颈前或后、委中、曲池。

【操作方法】

1. 先刮夹脊穴及其脊柱两侧的背俞穴区，重点刮拭心俞至肺俞，肾俞至腰俞区间，以皮肤潮红为度。

2. 再刮风池至肩井，至痧痕出现为止。

3. 合谷、太冲穴先点揉，再刮拭至皮肤泛红。

4. 根据病情刮拭配穴。颈前、后可用拧痧法；涌泉穴区可采用隔衣刮痧法，至局部皮肤温热感。

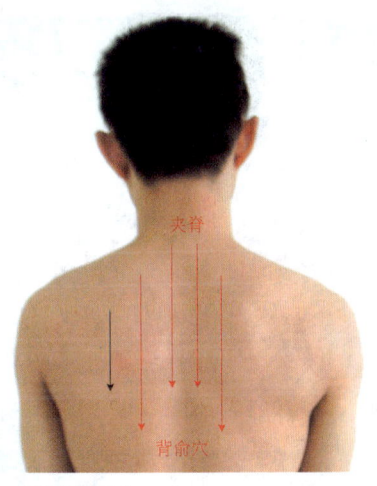

第九章　内科病症的刮痧疗法应用
Chapter 9 Guasha Therapy for Internal Diseases

图90 夹脊、背俞穴
Fig.90 Huatuo Jiaji (EX-B 2) points and back-Shu points

【注意事项】

1. 对于顽固性高血压或出现高血压危象者，应及时送医院就诊，采用中西医综合治疗方法，待病情稳定后再采用刮痧治疗。

2. 血压稳定后，可常直接刮拭或隔衣刮拭足三里、涌泉、太冲等穴以预防保健。

3. 注意调整饮食习惯，调节情绪，戒烟酒，节性欲，适当劳逸。

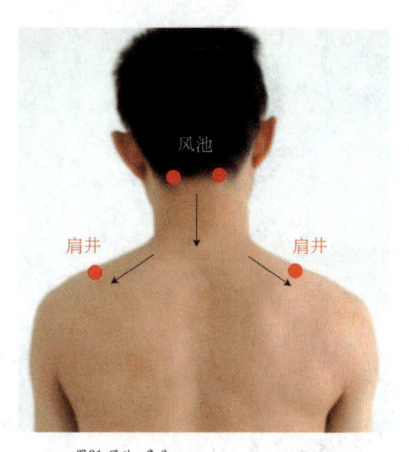

图91 风池、肩井
Fig.91 Fengchi (GB 20) and Jianjing (GB 21)

Section 14 Hypertension

Hypertension is one of the most common cardiovascular diseases. It is more common in the middle-aged and elderly. The primary clinical characteristic is increased arterial blood pressure, manifesting as increased systolic pressure or diastolic pressure or both, more specifically, the systolic pressure ≥140mmHg and diastolic pressure ≥90mmHg. Hypertension over a long period of time may affect the functions of key organs such as the heart, brain, and kidneys, leading to failure of organs, disability or even death. Traditional Chinese medicine asserts that factors such as the aging process, anxiety, intake of fatty or sweet food, mental stress, or intense irritation may play a role in the pathological process of hypertension.

[Major points] Huatuo Jiaji (EX-B 2) points, back-Shu points, Fengchi (GB 20), Jianjing (GB 21), Hegu (LI 4), and Taichong (LR 3). (See Fig.59, 71, 90-91)

[Point combination] For obesity due to phlegm-dampness resulting from fatty or sweet food, combine Baihui (GV 20), Fengfu (GV 16), Zusanli (ST 36), and Fenglong (ST 40); for deficiency of the liver and kidney due to the aging process, combine Sanyinjiao (SP 6), Taixi (KI 3), and Yongquan (KI 1); for irritability due to hyperactivity of fire in the liver and gallbladder, combine Toulinqi (GB 15), Fengchi (GB 20), Fengshi (GB 31), and Yanglingquan (GB 34); and if the patients does not respond well to the above methods, combine the neck or nape, Weizhong (BL 40), and Quchi (LI 11).

[Operation]

1. Scrape Jiaji (EX-B 2) points or back-Shu points first, especially from Xinshu (BL 15) to Feishu (BL 13) and from Shenshu (BL 23) to Yaoshu (GV 2) until the skin turns red.

2. Then scrape Fengchi (GB 20) down to Jianjing (GB 21) until Sha marks appear.

3. Knead Hegu (LI 4) and Taichong (LR 3) first and then scrape until the skin turns red.

4. Scrape other points according to specific symptoms, twist points in the neck or nape, and scrape Yongquan, with the socks on, until the patient feels warm in the local area.

[Cautionary notes]

1. Those with intractable hypertension or a hypertensive crisis need to go to hospital immediately for integrative Chinese-Western therapy. Guasha therapy can only be adopted after the patient's condition has stabilized.

2. When the patient's blood pressure has stabilized, scrape

Zusanli (ST 36), Yongquan (KI 1) and Taichong (LR 3), either directly or over the clothes to preserve health.

3. Regulate dietary habits, maintain a peaceful mind, cease smoking cigarettes or drinking alcohol, avoid sexual indulgence, and balance work and rest.

第十五节 面瘫

面瘫是以口眼歪斜为主要症状的一种疾病，表现为突然起病，每于睡醒后一侧面颊筋肉板滞、麻木、松弛、皱眉、额，耸鼻，鼓腮，吹气，露齿，闭眼等动作不能或不全，口角向健侧歪斜而无半身不遂、神志不清等症状。以春秋季多见，多见于20～40岁，男性略多。相当于现代医学的周围性面瘫。

【主穴】翳风、风池、颊车、颧髎、四白、阳白、合谷。（图58、59、92、93）

【配穴】鼻中沟歪斜配水沟、迎香；颏唇沟歪斜配承浆、地仓；目不能合配攒竹、丝竹空；耸鼻不能配迎香、鼻通；病程长者配足三里、三阴交。

【操作方法】

1. 以较重的力度刮拭主穴，以皮肤出现痧痕为度。

2. 根据病情刮拭配穴。

【注意事项】

1. 刮痧治疗期间可适当配合针灸推拿、热敷理疗。

2. 对于患侧眼睛干燥者可配合外用眼药水，防治感染。必要时需戴眼罩予以保护。

3. 注意避免患侧再次受凉，必要时外出可戴口罩予以保护。

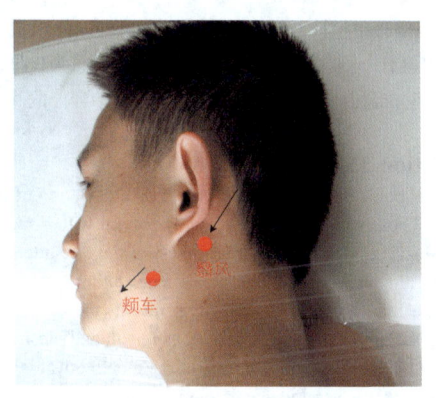

第九章 内科病症的刮痧疗法应用
Chapter 9 Guasha Therapy for Internal Diseases

图92 翳风、颊车
Fig.92 Yifeng (SJ 17) and Jiache (ST 6)

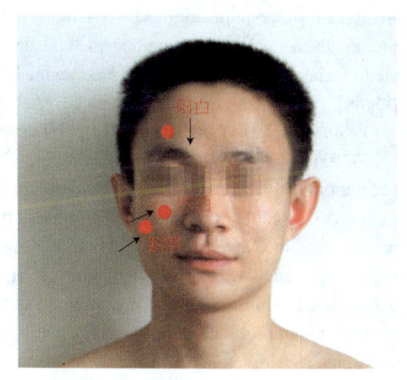

图93 阳白、四白、颧髎
Fig.93 Yangbai (GB 14), Sibai (ST 2), and Quanliao (SI 18)

4. 面瘫有中枢性与周围性之分。中枢性面瘫仅眼以下部位瘫痪，但伴有一侧肢体无力或瘫痪；周围性面瘫为口眼歪斜，无其他肢体功能异常。应注意鉴别，以免延误治疗，危及生命。

Section 15 Facial palsy

Facial palsy is mainly characterized by a deviation of the mouth and eyes. Those with facial palsy usually present with a sudden onset, one sided stiffness, numbness or looseness of the face after waking up in the morning. The patients will experience either a total loss of, or incomplete movement when frowning, raising the eyebrows, lifting the nose, puffing the cheeks, exposing the teeth and closing the eyes. There will be deviation of the corner of the mouth towards the healthy side, but with no hemiplegia or clouding of consciousness. Facial palsy mostly affects people around 20-40 years old and is more common in men than women. In addition, it is more common in spring and autumn. Facial palsy, as described in this section is the same as peripheral facial palsy (Bell's palsy) in modern medicine.

[Major points] Yifeng (SJ 17), Fengchi (GB 20), Jiache (ST 6), Quanliao (SI 18), Sibai (ST 2), Yangbai (GB 14), and Hegu (LI 4). (See Fig.58, 59, 92, 93)

[Points combination] For deviation of the nasolabial groove, combine Shuigou (GV 26) and Yingxiang (LI 20); for deviation of the mentolabial groove, combine Chengjiang (CV 24) and Dicang (ST 4); for an inability to close one's eyes, combine Cuanzhu (BL 2) and Sizhukong (SJ 23); for an inability to lift nose, combine Yingxiang (LI 20) and Bitong (Extra); and for a chronic condition, combine Zusanli (ST 36) and Sanyinjiao (SP 6).

[Operation]
1. Scrape major points with heavy force until Sha marks appear.
2. Scrape other joints according to specific symptoms.

[Cautionary notes]
1. Combine acupuncture, tuina, hot compression or physiotherapy during Guasha therapy.
2. Combine eye drops for those with dry eyes to prevent infection or suggest wearing an eyeshade to protect the eyes.
3. Avoid re-attack of cold to the affected side and wear a mask if necessary.
4. Peripheral facial palsy should be differentiated from central facial palsy first before commencing Guasha therapy. Those with peripheral facial palsy usually present with deviation of the mouth and eyes but with no dysfunction of limbs. However, those with central facial palsy may present with paralysis of the lower half of the face and complications of one sided weakness or hemiplegia.

第十六节　三叉神经痛

三叉神经痛是指三叉神经分布区内（三叉神经第一支，主要分布于额部；第二支主要分布于颧、面颊部；第三支主要分布于下颌）反复出现阵发性的剧烈疼痛，疼痛呈发作性闪电、刀割、针刺、烧灼样，持续数秒或数分钟，间歇期无症状，常因说话、吞咽、刷牙、洗脸等再次诱发。中医学认为本病多因感受风寒、风热外邪或肝胃郁火或阴虚火旺而导致。临床上40岁以上女性多见，以第二支和第三支发病为多。

【主穴】四白、下关、风池、合谷、太冲。（图59、71、93、94)

【配穴】上颌痛配颧髎；下颌痛配颊车；前额痛配阳白、攒竹；感受风寒配翳风；肝胃火旺配内庭；阴虚配三阴交、太溪。

【操作方法】

1. 以较重的力度从风池向下刮拭至肩井，直至痧痕出现。

2. 四白、列缺、合谷穴先点揉，再刮拭，也以痧痕出现为度。

3. 根据病症刮拭配穴。

【注意事项】

1. 三叉神经痛有原发性和继发性两种。对于继发性三叉神经痛需探明原因，及时采取适当措施，治疗原发病。

2. 注意饮食起居的调节。

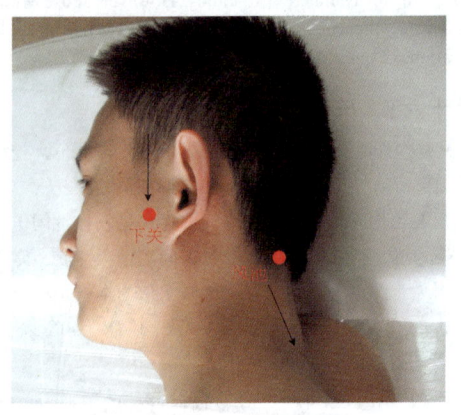

图94 下关、风池
Fig.94 Xiaguan (ST 7) and Fengchi (GB 20)

Section 16 Trigeminal neuralgia

Trigeminal neuralgia refers to the paroxysmal, severe headache within the distribution area of trigeminal nerve (the first branch mainly distributes over the forehead; the second branch over the zygomatic area and cheek; and the third branch over the lower mandible). The pain can be that of an electric shock, cutting, stabbing, or burning, lasting from seconds to minutes. No symptoms occur during intermission of pain. However, the pain can be induced by movements such as talking, swallowing, brushing one's teeth or washing one's face. Traditional Chinese medicine asserts that trigeminal neuralgia results from the following etiological factors: external contraction of wind-cold or wind-heat, stagnant fire in the liver and stomach, or hyperactivity of fire due to yin deficiency. It is more common in women above 40 years old, especially involving the 2nd and 3rd branches.

[Major points] Sibai (ST 2), Xiaguan (ST 7), Fengchi (GB 20), Hegu (LI 4), and Taichong (LR 3) .(See Fig.59, 71, 93, 94)

[Point combination] For pain in the upper jaw, combine Quanliao (SI 18); for pain in the lower mandible, combine Jiache (ST 6); for forehead pain, combine Yangbai (GB 14) and Cuanzhu (BL 2); for external contraction of wind-cold, combine Yifeng (SJ 17); for hyperactivity of fire in the liver and stomach, combine Neiting (ST 44); and for yin deficiency, combine Sanyinjiao (SP 6) and Taixi (KI 3).

[Operation]

1. Scrape from Fengchi (GB 20) down to Jianjing (GB 21) with a heavy force until Sha marks appear.

2. Knead Sibai (ST 2), Lieque (LU 7), and Hegu (LI 4) first and then scrape until Sha marks appear.

[Cautionary notes]

1. Trigeminal neuralgia can be primary or secondary. For secondary type, the true cause must be identified for appropriate treatment.

2. Regulate one's lifestyle.

第十章　骨伤外科病症的刮痧疗法应用

第一节　落枕

落枕是指突然颈项强痛，酸胀且活动受限的一种病症。常于晨起时发现。本病常因体虚劳累过度，睡姿不当，枕头高低不适使颈部肌肉维持长时间的过分牵拉或紧张状态而痉挛或因颈部扭伤或感受风寒，使筋脉气血阻滞而诱发。多见于成年人。若反复发作，常常是颈椎病变的反映。

【主穴】患侧风池、肩井、风门、天宗、落枕穴。（图91、95、96）

【配穴】外感风寒配外关；颈椎病配后溪、悬钟。

【操作方法】

1. 先刮患侧风池至肩井穴区，再刮风池、风门穴，至出现痧痕为止。

2. 天宗、落枕穴先点揉至酸胀感，再刮拭，以痧痕出现为度。

3. 可根据病情加刮配穴。

【注意事项】

1. 落枕刮痧治疗的同时可配合推拿疗法，效果较佳。

2. 平日应注意局部保暖，勿过度疲劳，避免再受风寒。注意调整睡姿。

3. 可配合作颈部健身操，即适度的前屈后仰、左旋右转、体转耸肩、迅速沉肩，每日3~4次。

下篇　刮痧疗法的实践应用
Part B Guasha Therapy in Practice

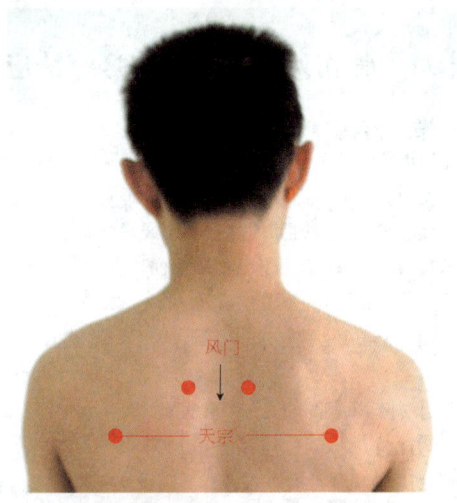

图95 风门、天宗
Fig.95 Fengmen (BL 12) and Tianzong (SI 11)

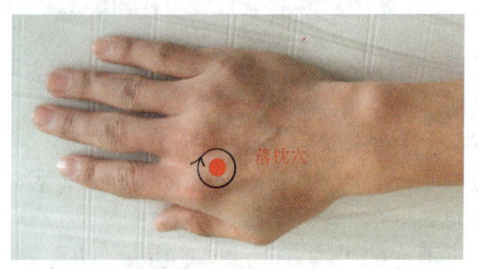

图96 落枕穴
Fig.96 Luozhen (Extra)

Chapter 10 Guasha Therapy for Traumatology and External Conditions

Section 1 Stiff neck

Stiff neck refers to sudden neck rigidity, pain, soreness and distension as well as limited movement. It occurs in the morning after getting up due to numerous factors. Fatigue, an improper sleeping posture or an uncomfortable pillow may cause over-extension or tension and spasm of the neck muscles. Cervical sprain or external contraction of wind-cold may also cause stagnation of qi and blood in the cervical area. Stiff neck is more common in adults. Frequent occurrence of stiff neck can be a precursor to cervical spondylosis.

[Major points] Fengchi (GB 20), Jianjing (GB 21), Fengmen (BL 12), and Tianzong (SI 11) of the affected side as well as Luozhen (Extra). (See Fig.91, 95, 96)

[Point combination] For external contraction of wind-cold, combine Waiguan (SJ 5); and for cervical spondylosis, combine Houxi (SI 3) and Xuanzhong (GB 39).

[Operation]

1. Scrape from Fengchi (GB 20) to Jianjing (GB 21) on the affected side, and then scrape Fengchi (GB 21) and Fengmen (BL 12) until Sha marks appear.

2. Knead Tianzong (SI 11) and Luozhen (Extra) until the patient feels soreness and distension, and then scrape until Sha marks appear.

3. Scrape other points according to specific symptoms.

[Cautionary notes]

1. Combine tuina therapy with Guasha treatment.

2. Keep the cervical area warm, avoid fatigue and wind-cold and be conscious of the sleeping posture.

3. Do neck exercises, for example, moderate anteflexion and posterior extension, left-right rotation, trunk rotation, shoulder shrugging with sudden shoulder relaxation, 3-4 times each day.

第二节 颈椎病

颈椎病,是颈椎综合征的简称。是由于增生性颈椎炎、颈椎间盘脱出,以及颈椎间关节、韧带等组织的退行性病变刺激或压迫颈神经根、脊髓、椎动脉和颈部交感神经等而出现的一组症候群。临床表现以颈项、肩臂、肩胛上部、上胸壁及上肢疼痛或麻痹,甚至颈部活动时出现眩晕等为主要特征。

【主穴】风池、肩井、膈俞、阳陵泉、悬钟、颈部夹脊穴区。(图97~99)

【配穴】上肢疼痛或麻痹配肩髃、曲池、外关;颈部转侧困难配后溪、承山;颈背酸痛配列缺、天宗;体虚者配足三里。

【操作方法】

1. 先重刮颈部夹脊穴区,风池至肩井,上背部肩胛内侧区,直至瘀痕出现为止。

2. 以中等力度刮拭阳陵泉至悬钟穴区,也以瘀痕出现为度。

3. 根据临床病证的表现,加刮配穴。

【注意事项】

1. 刮痧疗法对于神经根型的颈椎病疗效较佳,对于脊髓型、椎动脉缺血型有一定的疗效。

2. 平时注意纠正不良的生活习惯、工作姿势，长期伏案工作或操作电脑的人应定时做颈部健身操，以放松局部肌肉。

3. 治疗期间可同时配服中草药制剂，如颈复康冲剂、壮骨关节丸等，以加强疗效。

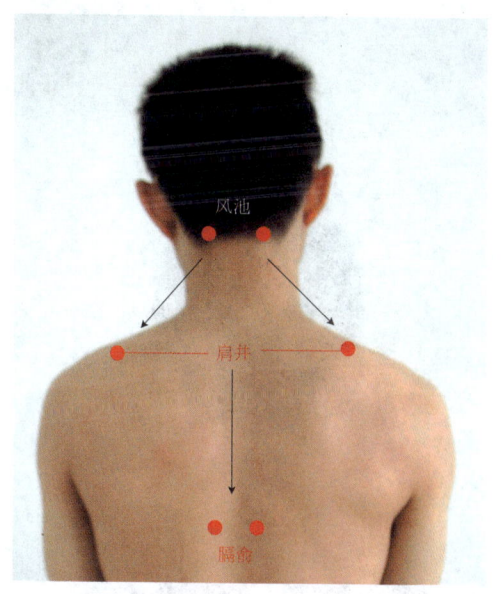

图97 风池、肩井、膈俞
Fig.97 Fengchi (GB 20), Jianjing (GB 21), and Geshu (BL 17)

下篇 刮痧疗法的实践应用
Part B Guasha Therapy in Practice

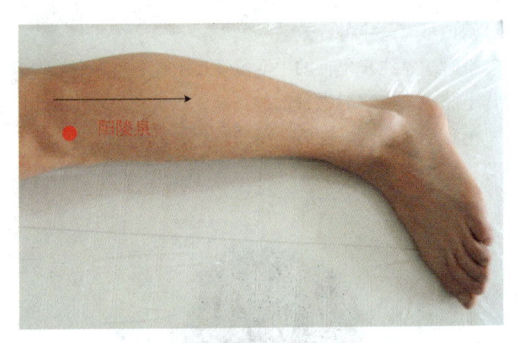

图98 阳陵泉
Fig.98 Yanglingquan (GB 34)

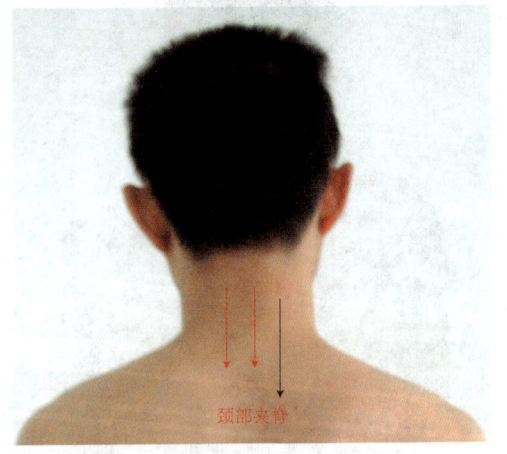

颈部夹脊

图99 颈部夹脊
Fig.99 Cervical Jiaji (EX-B 2) points

Section 2 Cervical spondylosis

Cervical spondylosis, also known as cervical spine syndrome, refers to a group of symptoms that result from proliferate cervical inflammation, herniation of cervical intervertebral discs or degeneration of intervertebral joints or ligaments. This causes compression of the cervical nerve root, spinal root, vertebral artery and cervical sympathetic nerve. This condition is characterized by pain or numbness in the neck or nape, shoulder, arm, suprascapular region, upper chest wall, and upper extremities. The patient may even experience vertigo upon neck movement.

[Major points] Fengchi (GB 20), Jianjing (GB 21), Geshu (BL 17), Yanglingquan (GB 34), Xuanzhong (GB 39), and cervical Jiaji (EX B 2) points . (See Fig.97-99)

[Point combination] For pain or numbness in the upper limbs, combine Jianyu (LI 15), Quchi (LI 11), and Waiguan (SJ 5); for difficulty in turning the neck to one side, combine Houxi (SI 3) and Chengshan (BL 57); for soreness and pain in the nape and back, combine Lieque (LU 7) and Tianzong (SI 11); and for those with a weak constitution, combine Zusanli (ST 36).

[Operation]

1, Scrape the cervical Jiaji (EX-B 2) points, Fengchi (GB 21) to Jianjing (GB 21), and the medial aspect of the scapula with a heavy force until Sha marks appear.

2. Scrape Yanglingquan (GB 34) to Xuanzhong (GB 29) with moderate force until the occurrence of Sha marks.

3. Scrape other points according to specific symptoms.

[Cautionary notes]

1. Guasha therapy works particularly well for nerve-root spondylosis and can help in cases of the spinal cord type or ischemic

vertebral artery type.

2. Maintain an appropriate lifestyle and correct working posture. Those with long-time sedentary jobs or long-term computer use should do cervical exercises regularly to relax the local muscles.

3. Combine Chinese herbal preparations such as Restoring Cervical Health Granules (jǐng fù kāng chōng jì) and Strengthening Bone and Joint Pill (zhuàng gǔ guān jié wán) to facilitate the therapeutic effect.

第三节 扭伤、劳损

扭伤、劳损是指近关节附近的软组织，如肌肉、肌腱、韧带、血管等损伤后痉挛、撕裂、瘀血肿胀，而无骨折、脱位、皮肤破损等的损伤症状。主要表现为局部肿胀、疼痛、关节活动受限。损伤部位常发生于各关节附近。

【主穴】天柱、肩井、大杼、膈俞。

肩部：肩髃、肩髎、肩贞、臑俞、阳陵泉。

肘部：曲池、曲泽、手三里。

腕部：阳池、阳溪、阳谷、外关。

腰部：肾俞、命门、腰眼、委中。

髋部：环跳、秩边、阳陵泉、委中。

膝部：梁丘、膝眼。

踝部：解溪、商丘、昆仑、丘墟。（图54、98、100~110）

【配穴】疼痛较重配太冲、合谷；瘀血胀甚者配血海、三阴交；局部红肿压痛明显配阿是穴，结合刺络拔罐。

【操作方法】

1. 重刮天柱至肩井、大杼至膈俞穴区,以痧痕出现为度。
2. 扭伤的部位选穴刮拭,直至皮肤出现痧痕为止。
3. 根据伴随症刮拭选穴。

【注意事项】

1. 注意排除骨折、脱位、韧带断裂等重症。
2. 新近扭伤的局部,应先以冰袋冷敷以防损伤处继续出血。
3. 新扭伤肿痛明显时,损伤周围刮痧手法宜轻,肿痛逐渐消退后可稍加重刮拭力度。

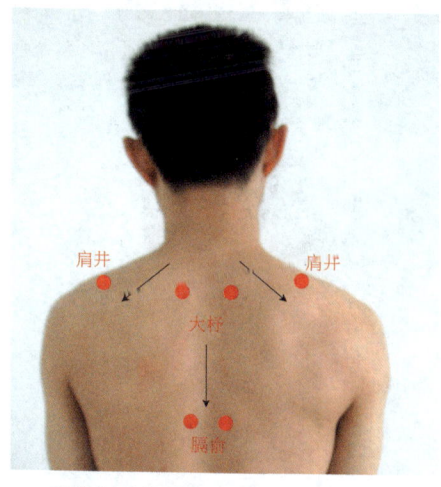

图100 肩井、大杼、膈俞
Fig.100 Jianjing (GB 21), Dazhu (BL 11), and Geshu (BL 17)

下篇 刮痧疗法的实践应用
Part B Guasha Therapy in Practice

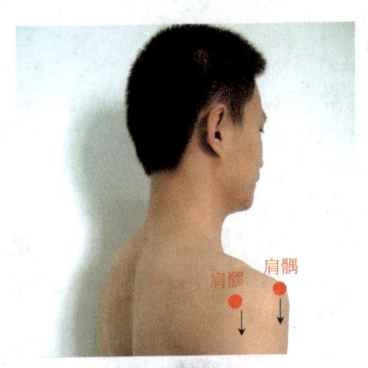

图101 肩髎、肩髃
Fig.101 Jianliao (SJ 14) and Jianyu (LI 15)

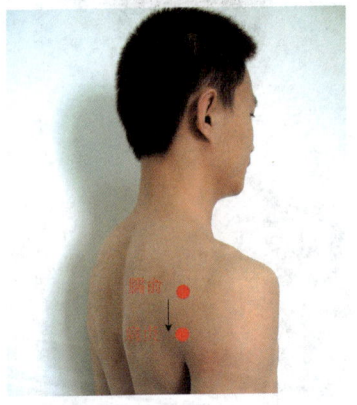

图102 臑俞、肩贞
Fig.102 Naoshu (SI 10) and Jianzhen (SI 9)

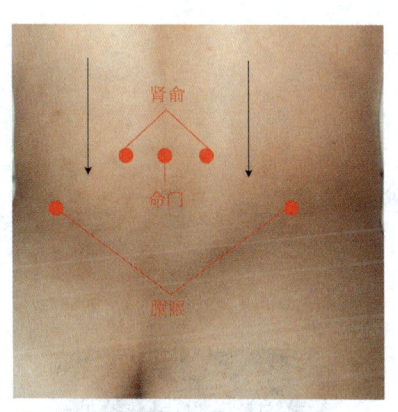

第十章 骨伤外科病症的刮痧疗法应用
Chapter 10 Guasha Therapy for Traumatology and External Conditions

图103 肾俞、命门、腰眼
Fig.103 Shenshu (BL 23), Mingmen (GV 4), and Yaoyan (EX-B 7)

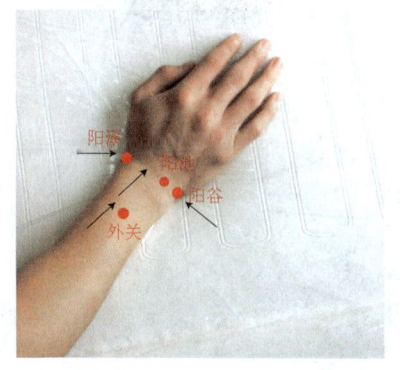

图104 外关、阳溪、阳池、阳谷
Fig.104 Waiguan (SJ 5), Yangxi (LI 5), Yangchi (SJ 4), and Yanggu (SI 5)

下篇　刮痧疗法的实践应用
Part B Guasha Therapy in Practice

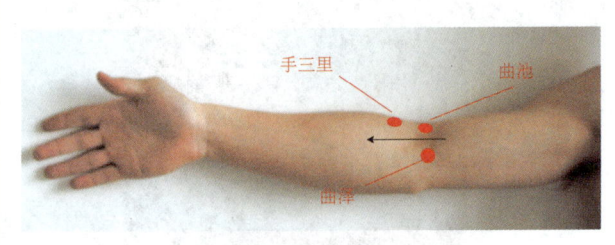

手三里
曲池
曲泽

图105 手三里、曲池、曲泽
Fig.105 Shousanli (LI 10), Quchi (LI 11), and Quze (PC 3)

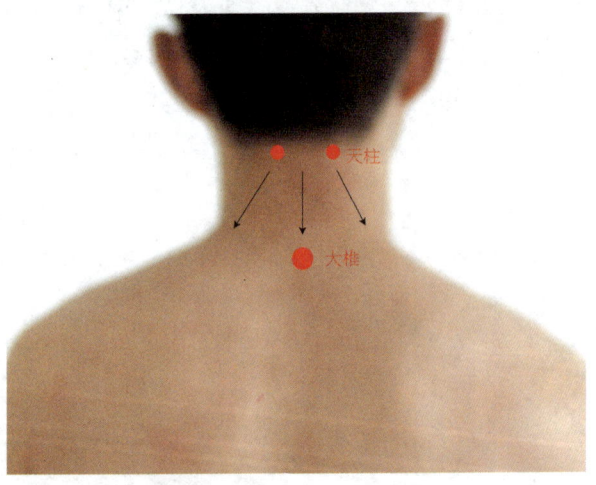

天柱
大椎

图106 天柱、大椎
Fig.106 Tianzhu (BL 10) and Dazhui (GV 14)

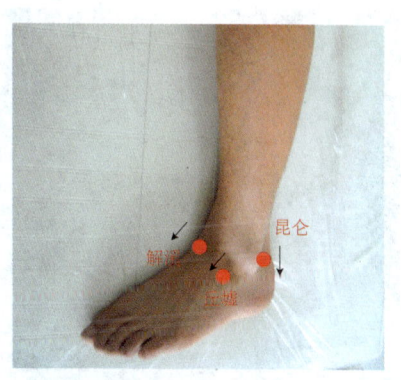

第十章 骨伤外科病症的刮痧疗法应用
Chapter 10 Guasha Therapy for Traumatology and External Conditions

图107 解溪、昆仑、丘墟
Fig.107 Jiexi (ST 41), Kunlun (BL 60), and Qiuxu (GB 40)

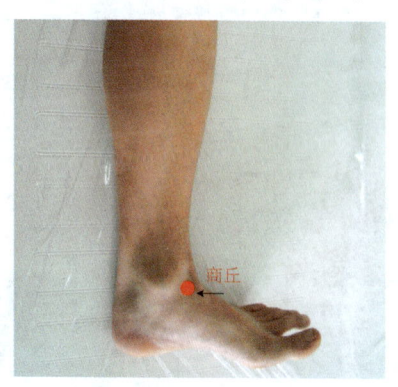

图108 商丘
Fig.108 Shangqiu (SP 5)

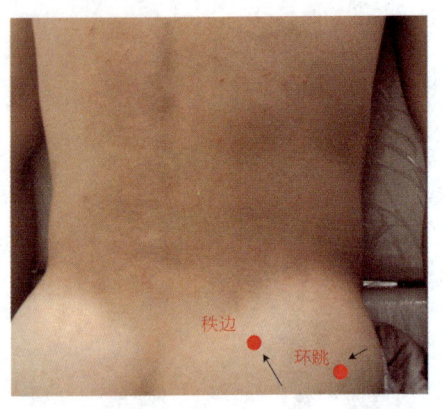

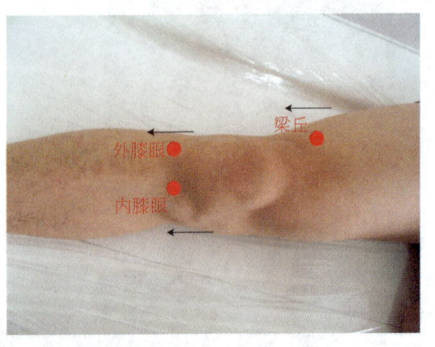

图109 秩边、环跳
Fig.109 Zhibian (BL 54) and Huantiao (GB 30)

图110 内膝眼、外膝眼、梁丘
Fig.110 Xiyan (EX–LE 5), Dubi (ST 35), and Liangqiu (ST 34)

Section 3 Sprain or strain

Sprain or strain refers to spasm, tearing or swelling of soft tissues adjacent to joints with resultant stagnant blood. The affected tissue may be muscle, tendon, ligament, or blood vessels but without traumatic symptoms such as fracture, dislocation or skin lesion. It mainly manifests as local swelling, pain, and limited movement. Lesions largely occurs in the areas around joints.

[Major points]

Tianzhu (BL 10), Jianjing (GB 21), Dazhu (BL 11), and Geshu (BL 17).

Shoulder area: Jianyu (LI 15), Jianliao (SJ 14), Jianzhen (SI 9), Naoshu (SJ 14) and Yanglingquan (GB 34).

Elbow area: Quchi (LI 11), Quze (PC 3), and Shousanli (LI 10).

Wrist area: Yangchi (SJ 4), Yangxi (LI 5), Yanggu (SI 5), and Waiguan (SJ 5).

Lumbar area: Shenshu (BL 23), Mingmen (GV 4), Yaoyan (EX-B 7), and Weizhong (BL 40).

Hip area: Huantiao (GB 30), Zhibian (BL 54), Yanglingquan (GB 34), and Weizhong (BL 40).

Knee area: Liangqiu (ST 34) and Xiyan (ST 35 or Extra).

Ankle area: Jiexi (ST 41), Shangqiu (SP 5), Kunlun (BL 60), and Qiuxu (GB 40) (See Fig.54, 98, 100-110).

[Point combination] For severe pain, combine Taichong (LR 3) and Hegu (LI 4); for distension due to stagnant blood, combine Xuehai (SP 10) and Sanyinjiao (SP 6); and for local swelling and tenderness, combine Ashi points and do cupping after blood-letting.

[Operation]

1. Scrape from Tianzhu (BL 10) to Jianjing (GB 21) and from Dazhu (BL 11) to Geshu (BL 17) with a heavy force until Sha marks

appear.

2. Scrape local points local to the sprained area until Sha marks appear.

3. Scrape other points according to specific symptoms

[Cautionary notes]

1. Severe conditions such as fracture, dislocation, and tearing of ligaments are contraindicated.

2. Apply an ice pack to the local area in an acute sprain to prevent continuous bleeding.

3. For significant swelling and pain upon acute injury, scrape the injured area with a mild force and only scrape with a slightly heavier force after the disappearance of swelling and pain.

第四节　肩凝证

肩凝证又称为"漏肩风"。是以单侧或双侧肩关节酸重疼痛、活动受限为主症。50岁左右女性多发，又称"五十肩"。日久不愈者可出现肩关节不同程度的僵直，上臂上举、外旋、外展、后伸等活动受限，甚至患部肌肉萎缩。

【主穴】肩井、缺盆、肩髃、秉风、天宗、曲池、外关、阿是穴（痛点）。（图56、91、111、112）

【配穴】肩后外侧疼痛明显配肩贞、条口、承山；肩前内侧疼痛明显配肩内陵、臂臑。

【操作手法】

1. 肩井、秉风、天宗、曲池、外关、阿是穴，先点按至酸胀，再以较重的力度刮拭，方向朝向肩关节。直至痧痕出现。

2. 再根据症候刮拭配穴。

【注意事项】

1. 坚持肩关节适当的运动（外旋、内旋、前屈、外展、后伸），以松解粘连、滑利关节，并伸展局部挛缩的肌腱、韧带。

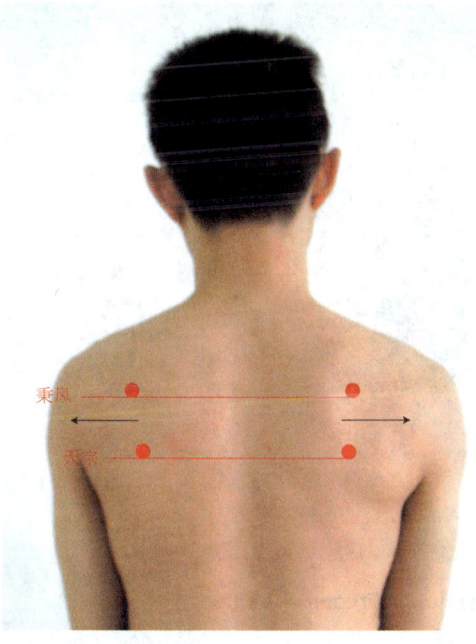

图111 秉风、天宗
Fig.111 Bingfeng (SI 12) and Tianzong (SI 11)

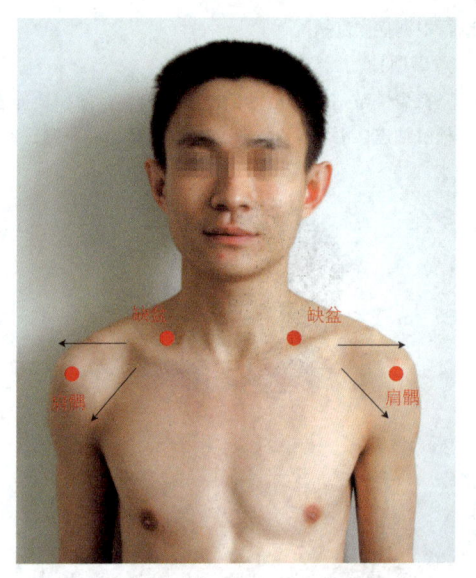

图112 缺盆、肩髃
Fig.112 Quepen (ST 12) and Jianyu (LI 15)

2. 应注意功能锻炼时动作宜轻宜缓，以患侧肩关节的能动幅度和患者的耐受能力为度。

3. 配合局部的热敷理疗。注意局部的保暖防寒。

Section 4 Frozen shoulder

Frozen shoulder, also known as 'leakage of shoulder wind' in traditional Chinese medicine, is mainly characterized by unilateral or bilateral soreness, heaviness, pain and limited movement of the shoulder joint. Since it is more common in women around 50 years old, it is also called 'shoulder of the 50 years old'. Long-term frozen shoulder may cause stiffness of the shoulder joint and limited movement, particularly in lifting up the upper arm, either in external rotation, abduction or posterior extension. There may even be muscle atrophy in the affected area.

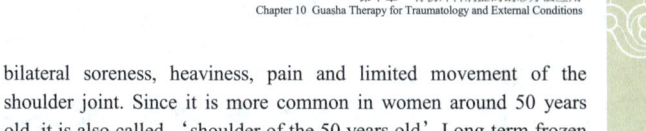

[Major points] Jianjing (GB 21), Quepen (ST 12), Jianyu (LI 15), Bingfeng (SI 12), Tianzong (SI 11), Quchi (LI 11), Waiguan (SJ 5), and Ashi points (tenderness spots) (See Fig.56, 91, 111, 112)

[Point combination] For significant pain in the posterior and lateral aspects of the shoulder, combine Jianzhen (SI 9), Tiaokou (ST 38) and Chengshan (BL 57); for significant pain in the anterior and medial aspects of the shoulder, combine Jianneiling (Extra), and Binao (LI 14).

[Operation]

1. Knead points Jianjing (GB 21), Bingfeng (SI 12), Tianzong (SI 11), Quchi (LI 11), Waiguan (SJ 5) and Ashi points until the patient feels soreness and distension. Then scrape towards the shoulder joint with a heavy force until Sha marks appear.

2. Scrape other points according to specific symptoms.

[Cautionary notes]

1. Do appropriate exercise of the shoulder joint (external rotation, internal rotation, abduction, and posterior extension) to release adhesion and lubricate joints, this will also extend the contractural tendons and ligaments of the local area.

2. Do functional exercises slowly and gently within the patient's tolerance and movement amplitude of the affected shoulder joint.

3. Combine hot compression and keep the local area warm.

第五节 腰痛

腰痛又称"腰脊痛"。指患者自觉腰部脊中、一侧或两侧疼痛的病证。多由于感受寒湿外邪或陈伤宿疾、腰部劳损或因年老体衰或久病劳欲，肾虚腰痛所致。

【主穴】腰阳关、肾俞、腰眼、委中、阿是穴。（图54、103、113）

【配穴】腰部酸痛、俯仰困难、因气候改变而发作的寒湿腰痛配次髎、阴陵泉、腰痛点、三阴交；劳损配次髎、秩边、膈俞、带脉、环跳；肾虚腰痛配命门、志室、三阴交、太溪。

【操作方法】

1. 腰阳关、肾俞、腰眼、委中先点按至酸胀，再刮拭，直至皮肤出现痧痕。

2. 根据病症辨证的不同，加刮配穴，寒湿、劳损腰痛应重刮；肾虚腰痛刮拭力度应轻柔。腰痛点可用点揉法。

【注意事项】

1. 腰痛治疗前应明确诊断，对于因脊椎结核、肿瘤、椎旁脓肿等引

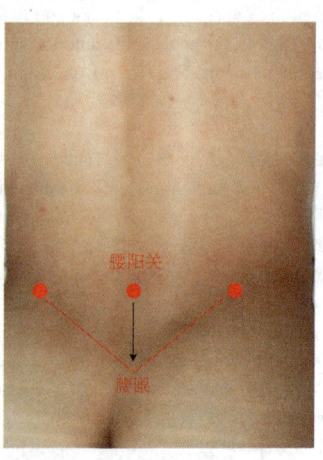

图113 腰阳关、腰眼
Fig.113 Yaoyangguan (GV 3) and Yaoyan (EX-B 7)

起的腰痛，应及时治疗原发病证。

2. 局部疼痛部位可配合热敷理疗。

3. 注意保暖防寒，调节生活起居，减轻腰痛并防止复发。

Section 5 Lower back pain

Lower back pain, also known as 'lumbar vertebra pain', refers to the subjective feeling of pain in the lumbar vertebra, and on the unilateral or bilateral sides of the lumbar vertebrae. It is caused by factors such as external contraction of cold-dampness, unresolved trauma, lumbar strain, a weak constitution due to the aging process, or kidney deficiency due to fatigue or sexual indulgence.

[Major points] Yaoyangguan (GV 3), Shenshu (BL 23), Yaoyan (EX-B 7), Weizhong (BL 40), and Ashi points. (See Fig.54, 103, 113)

[Point combination] For lumbar soreness and pain, difficulty in bending down, increased pain with weather changes, combine Ciliao (BL 32), Yinlingquan (SP 9), Yaotongdian (EX-UE 7), and Sanyinjiao (SP 6); for strain, combine Ciliao (BL 32), Zhibian (BL 54), Geshu (BL 17), Daimai (GB 26), and Huantiao (GB 30); and for lower back pain due to kidney deficiency, combine Mingmen (GV 4), Zhishi (BL 52), Sanyinjiao (SP 6), and Taixi (KI 3)

[Operation]

1. Knead points Yaoyangguan (GV 3), Shenshu (BL 23), Yaoyan (EX-B 7) and Weizhong (BL 40) until the patient feels soreness and distension, and then scrape until Sha marks appear.

2. Scrape other points according to specific symptoms, use a heavier force for lower back pain due to cold-dampness and strain, use a gentle force for lower back pain due to kidney deficiency, and knead Yaotongdian (EX-UE 7).

[Cautionary notes]

1. Be clear about the diagnosis of lower back pain and treat the primary cause such as vertebral tuberculosis, tumor or paravertebral abscess.

2. Combine hot compression for local pain.

3. Keep warm and regulate lifestyle to relieve lower back pain and prevent recurrence.

第六节　坐骨神经痛

坐骨神经痛是指坐骨神经通路的任何一段或全程出现放射性疼痛。临床以臀部、大腿后侧、小腿后外侧及足部放射性、烧灼样或针刺样疼痛等症候为主要特征。本病有原发性和继发性之分。前者多与感受风寒湿外邪，或劳损等因素有关，后者多因神经通路的邻近组织病变引发，如腰椎间盘脱出、脊椎肿瘤、腰骶部各关节或软组织损伤等。

【主穴】腰骶部夹脊穴、肾俞、腰眼、秩边、环跳、阿是穴（痛点）。（图103、109、114）

【配穴】原发性坐骨神经痛配血海、风市、阳陵泉；继发性配承扶、殷门、委中、承山；寒湿重配阴陵泉、地机、三阴交；有劳损病史者配次髎、膈俞、带脉；肾虚腰痛配命门、腰阳关、三阴交、太溪、志室。

【操作方法】

1. 腰骶部夹脊穴自上而下，由轻至重刮拭。腰眼、秩边、环跳、阿是穴等先点揉按至局部酸痛，再行刮痧，均以痧痕出现为度。

2. 再根据病情刮拭配穴。

【注意事项】

1. 对于因腰椎间盘脱出、脊椎肿瘤、椎旁脓肿或骨盆病变等引起的继发性坐骨神经痛,应明确诊断,及时治疗原发病或采取综合治疗。

2. 疼痛部位可配合热敷理疗,并注意保暖防寒,调节生活起居以免复发。

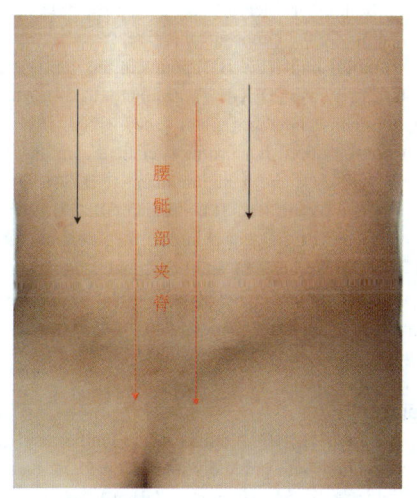

图114 腰骶部夹脊
Fig.114 Jiaji (EX-B 2) points in lumbosacral region

Section 6 Sciatica

Sciatica refers to radiating pain that occurs along either part of or the length of the sciatic nerve. It is clinically characterized by radiating, burning, or needle-pricking pain in the buttock, posterior aspect of the thigh, posterior and lateral aspect of the lower leg, and foot. Sciatica can be primary and secondary to other conditions. Primary sciatica is associated with external contraction of wind, cold, and dampness or strain. Secondary sciatica is often associated with pathology of the tissues adjacent to the nerve pathway such as herniation of the lumbar intervertebral disc, vertebral tumor, or joint or soft tissue injury in the lumbosacral region.

[Major points] Jiaji (EX-B 2) points in the lumbosacral region, Shenshu (BL 23), Yaoyan (EX-B 7), Zhibian (BL 54), Huantiao (GB 30), and Ashi points (tenderness spots). (See Fig.103, 109, 114)

[Point combination] For primary sciatica, combine Xuehai (SP 10), Fengshi (GB 31), and Yanglingquan (GB 34); for secondary sciatica, combine Chengfu (BL 36), Yinmen (BL 37), Weizhong (BL 40), and Chengshan (BL 57); for pain due to cold-dampness, combine Yinlingquan (SP 9), Diji (SP 8), and Sanyinjiao (SP 6); for those with history of strain, combine Ciliao (BL 32), Geshu (BL 17), and Daimai (GB 26); and for pain due to kidney deficiency, combine Mingmen (GV 4), Yaoyangguan (GV 3), Sanyinjiao (SP 6), Taixi (KI 3), and Zhishi (BL 52).

[Operation]

1. Scrape Jiaji (EX-B 2) points in the lumbosacral region in a downwards direction with gradually increasing force. Knead Yaoyan (EX-B 7), Zhibian (BL 54), Huantiao (GB 30), and Ashi points until the patient feels soreness and pain in the local area and then scrape until Sha marks appear.

2. Scrape other points according to specific symptoms.

[Cautionary notes]

1. Be clear about the diagnosis and treat the primary cause such as herniation of lumbar intervertebral disc, vertebral tumor, paravertebral abscess, or pelvic conditions.

2. Combine a hot compression for local pain, keep warm, and regulate the lifestyle to prevent recurrence.

第七节 网球肘

网球肘，即"肱骨外上髁炎"，是指因前臂旋转用力不当，或感受风寒湿，或劳损导致肘关节肱骨外上髁炎症，出现以肘关节外侧疼痛、用力握拳及前臂旋转动作如拧毛巾时疼痛加剧为特征的病症。

【主穴】肘髎、手三里、外关、阿是穴（痛点）。（图115）

【配穴】前臂旋转不当配肘窝、臑会；感受风寒湿配风池、肩井；劳损配大杼、膏肓俞、阳陵泉。

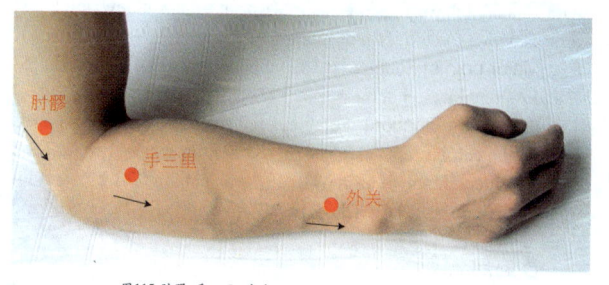

图115 肘髎、手三里、外关
Fig.115 Zhouliao (LI 12), Shousanli (LI 10), and Waiguan (SJ 5)

【操作方法】

1. 先刮阿是穴，至痧痕出现为止。

2. 肘髎至手三里、外关向腕关节方向以中等力度刮拭，至痧痕为度。

3. 根据病情刮拭配穴，以皮肤泛红为度。

【注意事项】

1. 注意用力得当，局部刺激强度不宜过量。

2. 治疗期间嘱患者应尽量减少肘部活动，更不易过劳，提取重物等。

3. 局部治疗可配合热敷理疗、针灸推拿等。

Section 7 Tennis elbow

Tennis elbow, also known as external humeral epicondylitis, is caused by factors such as inappropriate rotation of the forearm, external contraction of wind-cold, or strain. It is clinically characterized by pain in the lateral aspect of the elbow joint that worsens with a forceful grip or rotation of forearm.

[Major points] Zhouliao (LI 12), Shousanli (LI 10), Waiguan (SJ 5), and Ashi points (tenderness spots). (See Fig.115)

[Point combination] For impaired rotation of the forearm, combine the cubital fossa and Naohui (SJ 13); for external contraction of wind-cold, combine Fengchi (GB 20) and Jianjing (GB 21); and for strain, combine Dazhu (BL 11), Gaohuangshu (BL 43), and Yanglingquan (GB 34).

[Operation]

1. Scrape Ashi points first until Sha marks appear.

2. Scrape from Zhouliao (LI 12) to Shousanli (LI 10) and from Waiguan (SJ 5) to wrist joint with moderate force until the occurrence of Sha marks.

3. Scrape other points according to the specific symptoms until the skin turns red.

[Cautionary notes]

1. Use appropriate force and avoid too much stimulation to the local area.

2. Reduce elbow movement during course of treatment and avoid carrying heavy objects.

3. Combine a hot compression, tuina, or acupuncture in treating the local area.

第八节　腓肠肌痉挛

腓肠肌痉挛，又称为"腿肚转筋"。是指小腿肚的腓肠肌因受寒、过劳或外伤等引起突然抽搐、拘挛、疼痛为主要表现的病症。多在受凉后或游泳、劳作、夜间睡眠中发生。

【主穴】承山、阳陵泉、委中、申脉、昆仑。（图54、116、117）

【配穴】劳作或夜间发生者配三阴交、太溪、足三里、肾俞。

【操作方法】

1. 承山、阳陵泉、委中穴先点揉至局部酸胀感，再刮拭至痧痕出现。

2. 点按申脉、昆仑穴，以局部酸胀为度。

3. 根据病情刮拭其他配穴。

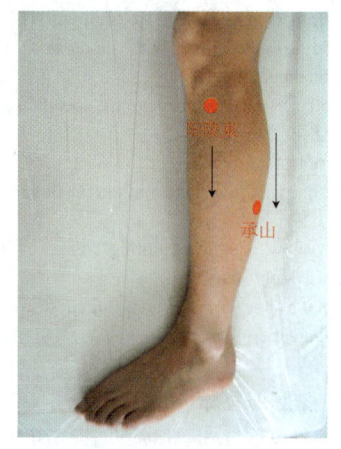

图116 阳陵泉、承山
Fig.116 Yanglingquan (GB 34) and Chengshan (BL 57)

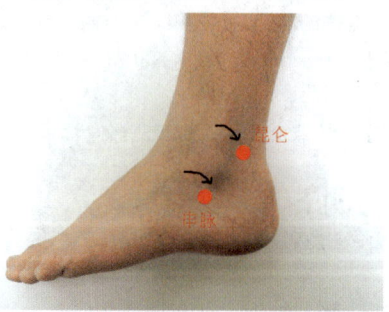

图117 昆仑、申脉
Fig.117 Kunlun (BL 60) and Shenmai (BL 62)

【注意事项】

1. 注意生活起居，忌食辛辣刺激食物，注意局部保暖，避免劳作过度。

2. 游泳中易发生腓肠肌痉挛者，应于游泳前做好热身运动，尤其注意揉搓局部。

3. 中老年人易发生痉挛者，可补充适量钙片或咨询专业医生以明确诊断。

Section 8 Sural spasm

Sural spasm, also known as 'calf muscle spasm', refers to sudden convulsion, contracture and pain in the gastrocnemius muscle. It can be caused by cold, strain or trauma and occurs upon attack of cold, swimming, physical work or during sleep.

[Major points] Chengshan (BL 57), Yanglingquan (GB 34), Weizhong (BL 40), Shenmai (BL 62), and Kunlun (BL 60). (See Fig. 54, 116, 117)

[Point combination] For sural spasm that occurs during physical work or sleep, combine Sanyinjiao (SP 6), Taixi (KI 3), Zusanli (ST 36), and Shenshu (BL 23).

[Operation]

1. Knead points Chengshan (BL 57), Yanglingquan (GB 34) and Weizhong (BL 40) until the patient feels soreness and distension and then scrape until Sha marks appear.

2. Knead Shenmai (BL 62) and Kunlun (BL 60) until the patient feels soreness and distension in the local area.

3. Scrape other points according to specific symptoms.

[Cautionary notes]

1. Regulate the lifestyle, stay away from spicy food, keep the local area warm, and avoid overstrain.

2. Do warm-up exercises before swimming by kneading or rubbing the local area.

3. Supplement calcium tablets or consult a specialist in cases of the elderly with frequent sural spasm.

第十一章 妇儿科病症的刮痧疗法应用

第一节 消化不良（食积）

消化不良（食积）多由于饮食不节或素体脾胃虚弱又饮食不当导致食物停骤不化、滞而不消的胃肠疾患。以饮食不思或食而不化、脘腹胀满疼痛、嗳气呕吐、大便酸臭或溏薄为特征。

【主穴】梁门、天枢、足三里、上巨虚、大肠俞、四缝。（图66、88、89、118、119）

【配穴】胃肠胀满疼痛配中脘、腹通谷、大横、梁丘；脾胃虚弱配脾俞、胃俞；呕吐配内关、合谷。

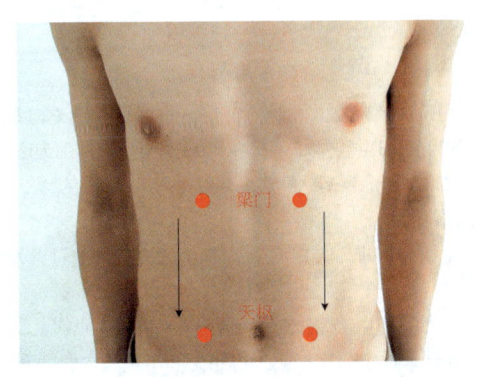

图118 梁门、天枢
Fig.118 Liangmen (ST 21) and Tianshu (ST 25)

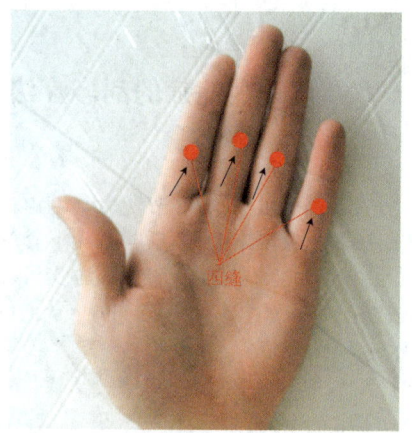

图119 四缝
Fig.119 Sifeng (EX-UE 10)

【操作方法】

1. 先刮梁门至天枢、大肠俞、足三里向踝关节方向刮拭,以皮肤泛红为度;四缝,取2~3处,以痧法至痧痕出现为度。

2. 再根据临床症候刮拭配穴。合谷、内关可用点揉法。

【注意事项】

1. 注意饮食调理,定时定量,避免过饱过饥或过食油腻、生冷食物。

2. 注意饮食卫生,预防各种肠道传染病和寄生虫病。

3. 小儿刮痧注意力度轻柔,应用柔和不刺激皮肤的刮痧介质,如油类为佳。皮肤以见微红为度。

Chapter 11 Guasha Therapy for Gynecological and Pediatric Conditions

Section 1 Dyspepsia (food retention)

Dyspepsia (food retention) is caused by either improper diet alone or combined with constitutional deficiency of the spleen and stomach. It is clinically characterized by a poor appetite, indigestion, gastric or abdominal fullness, distension, and pain, belching, vomiting, feces with foul breath, or loose stools.

[Major points] Liangmen (ST 21), Tianshu (ST 25), Zusanli (ST 36), Shangjuxu (ST 37), Dachangshu (BL 25), and Sifeng (EX-UE 10) .(See Fig.66, 88, 89, 118, 119)

[Point combination] For gastric fullness, distension, and pain, combine Zhongwan (CV 12), Futonggu (KI 20), Daheng (SP 15), and Liangqiu (ST 34); for deficiency of the spleen and stomach, combine Pishu (BL 20) and Weishu (BL 21); and for vomiting, combine Neiguan (PC 6) and Hegu (LI 4).

[Operation]

1. Scrape from Liangmen (ST 21) to Tianshu (ST 25), scrape Dachangshu (BL 25) and then scrape from Zusanli (ST 36) towards the ankle joints until the skin turns red; Select 2-3 points of Sifeng (EX-UE 10) and scrape until Sha marks appear.

2. Scrape other points according to specific symptoms. Knead Hegu (LI 4) and Neiguan (PC 6).

[Cautionary notes]

1. Maintain a regular diet, avoid hunger or overeating, and stay away from oily, raw, and cold food.

2. Maintain a high level of food to prevent enteric infectious diseases and parasitic diseases.

3. Use a gentle force and soft medium, such as oil, for children until slight redness appears.

第二节　百日咳

百日咳是感染百日咳杆菌引起的呼吸道传染病。以阵发性咳嗽，咳后伴有特殊吸气性吼声为特征。可持续2～3个月。以冬春季多发。多由于外感风寒、风热、疫邪，痰热壅肺，最后导致脾肺气虚。

【主穴】风池、风门、肺俞、天突、中府。（图58、67、120）

【配穴】寒咳配风池、肩井；痰热盛配尺泽、鱼际、曲池、丰隆；恢复期脾肺气虚配肺俞、膏肓俞、中脘、足三里、脾俞、肾俞、三阴交、太溪。

【操作方法】

1. 先从风池向下刮至大椎、风门至肺俞、天突至中府穴区，再刮拭上肢内侧前缘，直至皮肤泛红或至痧痕出现。

2. 根据病情辨证加刮配穴。

【注意事项】

1. 病情危重症及时送医院并配合药物综合治疗。

2. 发病期间应隔离，衣服用具等应煮沸消毒。保持环境安

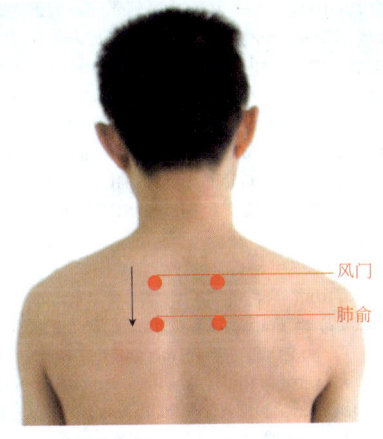

图120 风门、肺俞
Fig.120 Fengmen (BL 12) and Feishu (BL 13)

静、室内空气清新、温度适中。避免尘土异味刺激。

3. 注意按时接种百日咳疫苗。

Section 2 Whooping cough

Whooping cough is a type of respiratory infectious disease caused by the bacteria pertussis bacillus. It is identified by a paroxysmal cough and the subsequent characteristics aspiratory croup. Whooping cough may last 2-3 months and easily occurs in winter and spring. External contraction of wind-cold, wind-heat, or epidemic qi may cause accumulation of phlegm-heat in the lung, eventually resulting in qi deficiency of the spleen and lung and whooping cough.

[Major points] Fengchi (GB 20), Fengmen (BL 12), Feishu (BL 13), Tiantu (CV 22), and Zhongfu (LU 1) .(See Fig.58, 67, 120)

[Point combination] For cough due to cold, combine Fengchi (GB 20) and Jianjing (GB 21); for exuberance of phlegm-heat, combine Chize (LU 5), Yuji (LU 10), Quchi (LI 11), and Fenglong (ST 40); and for qi deficiency of the spleen and lung in the remission stage, combine Feishu (BL 13), Gaohuangshu (BL 43), Zhongwan (CV 12), Zusanli (ST 36), Pishu (BL 20), Shenshu (BL 23), Sanyinjiao (SP 6), and Taixi (KI 3).

[Operation]

1. Scrape from Fengchi (GB 20) to Dazhui (GV 14), from Fengmen (BL 12) to Feishu (BL 13), and Tiantu (CV 22) down to Zhongfu (LU 1), and then scrape the anterior border of the medial aspect of the upper arm until the skin turns red or Sha marks appear.

2. Scrape other points according to specific symptoms.

[Cautionary notes]

1. Those with life-threatening conditions should be sent to hospital immediately for comprehensive therapy.

2. Quarantine those with whooping cough, disinfest all the clothes and tools, keep the room quiet and fresh with a moderate temperature, and avoid contact with dust and flavorings.

3. Inoculate with the pertussis vaccine in good time.

第三节 痛经

痛经是指妇女随月经周期出现行经前后，或行经期间小腹部疼痛为特征的病症。以青少年女性多见。中医学认为，经期感寒饮冷或坐卧湿地，或情志不畅，肝郁气滞，或久病体虚等常是

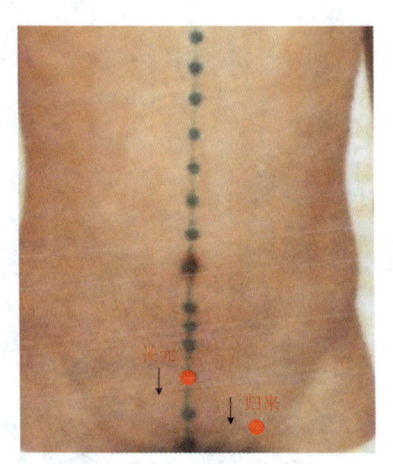

图121 关元、归来
Fig.121 Guanyuan (CV 4) and Guilai (ST 29)

痛经发生的原因。

【主穴】次髎、关元、归来、地机、三阴交。（图121～123）

【配穴】感受寒湿配命门、腰阳关、肾俞；肝郁气滞配太冲、膈俞、肝俞、期门；久病体虚配气海、关元、足三里。

【操作方法】

1. 次髎、地机、三阴交穴先点揉至酸胀感，再刮拭至痧痕出现。

2. 关元、归来穴向下刮拭，以皮肤泛红为度。

3. 再根据病情辨证刮拭配穴。

下篇　刮痧疗法的实践应用
Part B Guasha Therapy in Practice

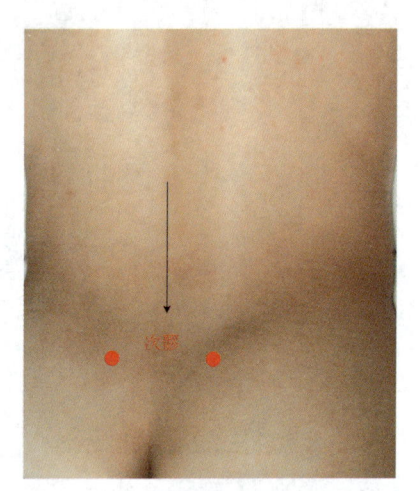

图122 次髎
Fig.122 Ciliao (BL 32)

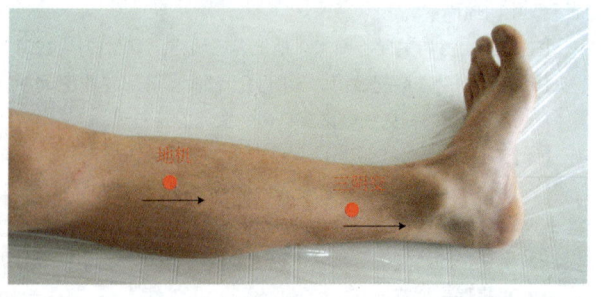

图123 地机、三阴交
Fig.123 Diji (SP 8) and Sanyinjiao (SP 6)

【注意事项】

1. 痛经诊治应探明病因，若因子宫内膜异位症、子宫肌瘤等应及时治疗原发病。

2. 注意调节经期或其前后的饮食起居。注意防寒保暖，忌食生冷。

Section 3 Dysmenorrhea

Dysmenorrhea refers to lower abdominal pain in women before, during, or after menstruation. It is more common in teenage girls. Traclitional Chinese medicine asserts that factors such as cold drinks, sitting or lying in wet places, liver-qi stagnation due to emotional distress, and a weak constitution due to chronic disease may play certain roles in dysmenorrhea.

[Major points] Ciliao (BL 32), Guanyuan (CV 4), Guilai (ST 29), Diji (SP 8), and Sanyinjiao (SP 6) (See Fig.121-123)

[Point combination] For external contraction of cold-dampness, combine Mingmen (GV 4), Yaoyangguan (GV 3), and Shenshu (BL 23); for liver-qi stagnation, combine Taichong (LR 3), Geshu (BL 17), Ganshu (BL 18), and Qimen (LR 14); and for a weak constitution due to chronic condieions, combine Qihai (CV 6), Guanyuan (CV 4), and Zusanli (ST 36).

[Operation]

1. Knead points Ciliao (BL 32), Diji (SP 8) and Sanyinjiao (SP 6) until the patient feels soreness and distension then scrape until Sha marks appear.

2. Scrape Guanyuan (CV 4) and Guilai (ST 29) downward until the skin turns red.

3. Scrape other points according to specific symptoms.

[Cautionary notes]

1. Be clear about the true cause of dysmenorrhea and treat the primary causes such as endometriosis and uterine fibrosis.

2. Regulate the lifestyle before, during, and after menstruation, keep warm, and stay away from raw and cold food.

第四节　月经不调

月经不调是以月经周期紊乱，出现经早、经迟或经乱1周以上，且伴有经量、色、质等异常及其他症状，并连续出现超过3个月经周期为主要表现的妇科病症。本病多因感受寒邪、忧思郁怒、情志失衡或劳倦体虚、房劳过度导致冲任失调或失养所致。因气候、环境、生活或情绪波动等引起月经周期的暂时改变（不超过3个月经周期者），不属于病态范畴。

【主穴】气海、关元、归来、三阴交。（图121、123、124）

【配穴】经早属血热者配大椎、血海、太冲、膈俞；经早属气虚配脾俞、肾俞、足三里、百会；经迟属肝郁气滞者配膈俞、肝俞、期门、太冲；血虚配膈俞、脾俞、血海、足三里；肾虚配肾俞、八髎穴区；血瘀配膈俞、血海、太冲、合谷。

【操作方法】

1. 气海、关元、归来刮向阴部毛际前，以皮肤潮红为度。

2. 三阴交先点按，再刮拭至皮肤潮红。

3. 根据病情不同刮拭配穴。

【注意事项】

1. 注意疾病的诊断，对于因垂体前叶病变或卵巢功能异常或肿瘤引起的，应及时治疗原发病。

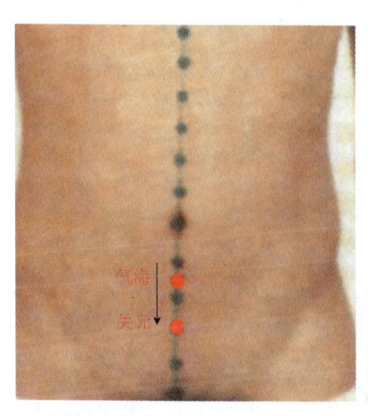

图124 关元、气海
Fig. 124 Guanyuan (CV 4) and Qihai (CV 6)

2. 注意经期及其前后饮食、起居、情志的调摄。
3. 可同时配服益母草膏等中成药。

Section 4 Irregular menstruation

Irregular menstruation is clinically characterized by 3 successive irregular menstrual cycles, more than 1 week early or delayed, irregular period, abnormal menstrual volume, color, and quality as well as other symptoms. Traditional Chinese medicine asserts that irregular menstruation is usually caused by disorder or malnutrition of Chong and Ren meridians due to factors including external contraction of cold, anxiety, emotional liability, fatigue or sexual indulgence. The temporary change of menstrual cycles (less than 3 months) due to weather, environment, life or emotional fluctuations is not considered a pathological condition.

[Major points] Qihai (CV 6), Guanyuan (CV 4), Guilai (ST 29), and Sanyinjiao (SP 6). (See Fig.121, 123, 124)

[Point combination] For an early period due to blood heat, combine Dazhui (CV 14), Xuehai (SP 10), Taichong (LR 3), and Geshu (BL 17); for an early period due to qi deficiency, combine Pishu (BL 20), Shenshu (BL 23), Zusanli (ST 36), and Baihui (GV 20); for a delayed period due to liver-qi stagnation, combine Geshu (BL 17), Ganshu (BL 18), Qimen (LR 14), and Taichong (LR 3); for blood deficiency, combine Geshu (BL 17), Pishu (BL 20), Xuehai (SP 10), and Zusanli (ST 36); for kidney deficiency, combine Shenshu (BL 23), and area of Baliao (bilateral BL 31-34); and for blood stasis, combine Geshu (BL 17), Xuehai (SP 10), Taichong (LR 3), and Hegu (LI 4).

[Operation]

1. Scrape from Qihai (CV 6), Guanyuan (CV 4), and Guilai (ST 29) downwards to the pubic hair until the skin turns red.

2. Knead Sanyinjiao (SP 6) first and then scrape until skin turns red.

3. Scrape other points according to specific symptoms

[Cautionary notes]

1. Take care to diagnose and treat the primary cause, such as pathology of the anterior lobule of pituitary, abnormal ovarian function, or tumor.

2. Regulate diet, lifestyle and emotions before, during and after menstruation.

3. Combine patent Chinese medicine such as Extractum leonuri Inspissatum (yì mǔ cǎo gāo).

第五节　乳腺小叶增生

常见于青、中年妇女。患者自觉乳房胀病或刺痛，兼有胸闷、嗳气等症状。一侧或两侧乳房发生多个大小不等的圆形结节。结节与周围组织分界不很清楚，结节可以推动。症状在行经前增加，行经后减轻，亦可因情志喜怒而消长。目前病因尚不清楚，可能与孕激素、雌激素的比例失衡有关。中医学认为多由郁怒、忧思，或冲任失调所致。

【主穴】屋翳、膻中、足三里、天宗、肩井、肾俞。（图63、66、91、95、125）

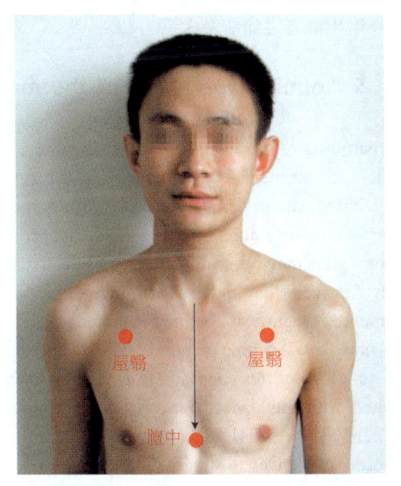

图125 屋翳、膻中
Fig.125 Wuyi (ST 15) and Danzhong (CV 17)

【配穴】肝郁配肝俞、太冲；血虚配血海、三阴交。

【操作方法】

1. 屋翳、膻中向下刮拭；足三里向小腿下方刮拭；肩井向肩峰刮拭；天宗向肩胛骨下缘刮拭；肾俞向腰部刮拭，均至皮肤潮红为度。

2. 根据病情常规刮拭配穴。

【注意事项】

1. 应保持情绪稳定，心情舒畅，忌辛辣煎炸之品。

2. 治疗前需明确诊断，对乳房纤维瘤经治疗后迅速增大者，或绝经期有慢性增生病者，均应考虑手术。

Section 5 Lobula hyperplasia of the mammary gland

Lobula hyperplasia of the mammary gland is more common in young to middle-aged women. The patients may subjectively feel distension or a stabbing pain in the breasts, along with symptoms such as chest stuffiness and belching. Multiple round-shaped, movable nodules in different sizes may occur unilaterally or bilaterally. There is no clear border between the nodules and peripheral tissue. The symptoms become more significant before the period and relieve after. The symptoms may also become better or worse upon emotional fluctuations. The etiology of this condition is as yet unknown yet. It is possibly associated with imbalanced ratio between progestogen and estrogen. It is believed in TCM to be related to depressed anger, anxiety or a disorder of the Chong and Ren meridians.

[Major points] Wuyi (ST 15), Danzhong (CV 17), Zusanli (ST

36), Tianzong (SI 11), Jianjing (GB 21), and Shenshu (BL 23). (See Fig.63, 66, 91, 95, 125)

[Point combination] For liver-qi stagnation, combine Ganshu (BL 18) and Taichong (LR 3); and for blood deficiency, combine Xuehai (SP 10) and Sanyinjiao (SP 6).

[Operation]

1. Scrape Wuyi (ST 15) and Danzhong (CV 17) downwards, scrape from Zusanli (ST 36) to the lower leg, scrape Jianjing (GB 21) towards the acromion; scrape Tianzong (SI 11) towards the inferior border of the scapula; and scrape Shenshu (BL 23) down to the lumbar region until the skin turns red.

2. Scrape other points according to specific symptoms.

[Cautionary notes]

1. Maintain a peaceful mind and stay away from spicy and fried food.

2. Be clear about the diagnosis and consider surgery for conditions such as a post-treatment rapid augmentation of mastofibroma or chronic hyperplasia during menopause.

第十二章 五官科病症的刮痧疗法应用

第一节 目赤肿痛

目赤肿痛是指以目赤、疼痛伴多泪或眼肿为主要表现的急性眼病。中医学认为，本病多因感受风热时邪或郁怒过度，肝胆火旺所致。

【主穴】攒竹、太阳、风池、合谷。（图58、59、69、126）

【配穴】风热时邪外感配大椎、三间；肝胆郁热配光明、悬

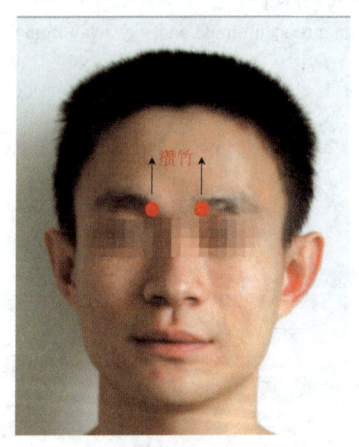

图 126 攒竹
Fig.126 Cuanzhu (BL 2)

钟、太冲、地五会。

【操作方法】

1. 太阳穴、攒竹、合谷点按至酸胀，再从攒竹向上刮拭、太阳穴向额角及耳尖前、合谷向示指方向刮拭至痧痕出现。

2. 风池穴向项后及肩部刮拭，也以痧痕出现为度。

3. 根据病情辨证刮拭配穴。

【注意事项】

1. 春秋季节常见本病传染，应注意隔离。

2. 注意平日保持眼部清洁卫生。

3. 必要时，可配合消炎眼药水外用。

Chapter 12　Guasha Therapy for Eye, Ear, Nose, and Throat Conditions

Section 1　Conjunctivitis

Conjunctivitis is an acute eye problem characterized by eye redness, eye pain with tears, and swelling of the eyes. According to traditional Chinese medicine, it can be caused by factors such as external contraction of wind-heat or hyperactivity of fire in the liver and gallbladder due to excessive anger.

[Major points] Cuanzhu (BL 2), Taiyang (EX-HN 5), Fengchi (GB 20), and Hegu (LI 4) .(See Fig.58, 59, 69, 126)

[Point combination] For external contraction of wind-heat, combine Dazhui (GV 14) and Sanjian (LI 3); and for stagnant heat in the liver and gallbladder, combine Guangming (GB 37), Xuanzhong (GB 39), Taichong (LR 3), and Diwuhui (GB 42).

[Operation]

1. Knead Taiyang (EX-HN 5), Cuanzhu (BL 2), and Hegu (LI 4) until the patient feels soreness and distension and then scrape Cuanzhu (BL 2) upwards, scrape Taiyang (EX-HN 5) towards the temples and area anterior to the ear apex, and scrape Hegu (LI 4) towards the index finger until Sha marks appear.

2. Scrape Fengchi (GB 20) towards the nape and shoulder until Sha marks appear.

3. Scrape other points according to specific symptoms.

[Cautionary notes]

1. Since it can be contagious in spring and autumn, those with conjunctivitis should be quarantined.

2. Keep the eyes clean.

3. Combine anti-inflammatory eye drops if necessary.

第二节 麦粒肿

麦粒肿，又称"睑腺炎"。是眼睑腺组织急性化脓性病症。临床上有发生于睫毛皮脂腺的外麦粒肿和睑板腺的内麦粒肿之分，多见于青少年。本病多因风邪外袭或嗜食辛辣煎炸之品而致脾胃湿热，忧思恼怒而致肝胆火旺引起。热毒蕴结或体质虚弱、屈光不正等常为本病反复发作的诱因。

【主穴】丝竹空、太阳、四白、风池。（图69、93、127）

【配穴】外感风热配外关、阳池、合谷；脾胃积热配合谷、曲池、阴陵泉；肝胆火旺配太冲、光明、悬钟、阳陵泉。

【操作方法】

1. 丝竹空、四白、太阳穴点按，丝竹空、四白分别刮向太阳穴，再从太阳穴呈扇形刮项、额角与耳尖前。

2. 风池穴刮向项后及肩部，以痧痕出现为度。

3. 根据临床辨证刮拭配穴，均以痧痕出现为度。

【注意事项】

1. 麦粒肿初期切忌挤压。成脓后应及时转眼科治疗。

2. 注意平日饮食起居的调节。忌食煎炸辛辣之品。

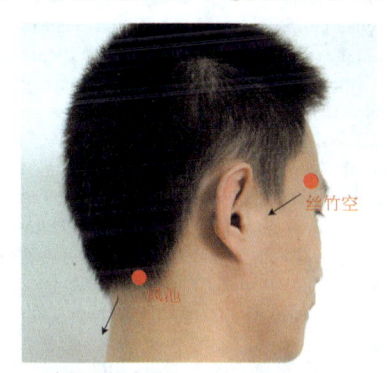

图127 丝竹空、风池
Fig.127 Sizhukong (SJ 23) and Fengchi (GB 20)

Section 2 Stye

A stye, also known as an 'inflammation of eyelid glands', is an acute purulent disorder of the glandular tissue of the eyelids. A stye can occur in the sebaceous gland of the eyelashes (external stye) or tarsal glands (internal stye). It is more common in teenagers. Traditional Chinese medicine asserts that a stye can be caused by factors such as damp-heat in the spleen and stomach due to wind attack or intake of spicy or fried food, or hyperactivity of fire in the liver and gallbladder due to anxiety and anger. The recurrence of a stye is triggered by toxic-heat accumulation, a weak constitution, or ametropia.

[Major points] Sizhukong (SJ 23), Taiyang (EX-HN 5), Sibai (ST 2), and Fengchi (GB 20) .(See Fig.69, 93, 127)

[Point combination] For external contraction of wind-heat, combine Waiguan (SJ 5), Yangchi (SJ 4), and Hegu (LI 4); for heat accumulating in the spleen and stomach, combine Hegu (LI 4), Quchi (LI 11), and Yinlingquan (SP 9); and for hyperactivity of fire in the liver and gallbladder, combine Taichong (LR 3), Guangming (GB 37), Xuanzhong (GB 39), and Yanglingquan (GB 34).

[Operation]

1. Knead Sizhukong (SJ 23), Sibai (ST 2) and Taiyang (EX-HN 5), then scrape Sizhukong (SJ 23) and Sibai (ST 2) towards Taiyang (EX-HN 5), and then scrape Taiyang (EX-HN 5) towards the temples and areas anterior to the ear apex.

2. Scrape Fengchi (GB 20) towards the nape and shoulder until Sha marks appear.

3. Scrape other points according to specific symptoms.

[Cautionary notes]

1. Avoid squeezing on early-stage stye and ophthalmology treatment is needed for purulence.

2. Regulate dietary habit and lifestyle and stay away from fried or spicy food.

第三节 牙痛

牙痛常因素体肠胃郁热，又嗜食辛辣煎炸或感受风热外邪，或年老体虚，虚火上扰，或口腔不洁、秽垢蚀齿而致，并常因冷、热、甜、酸等刺激而诱发。

【主穴】颊车、下关、合谷。（图59、128）

【配穴】风火牙痛配风池、外关、太阳；胃火牙痛配曲池、外关、内庭；便秘配左外关、左归来、左气冲；虚火牙痛配三阴交、太溪、行间、涌泉。

【操作方法】

1. 以中或重力度点按颊车、下关、合谷穴至局部酸胀，合谷穴向示指末端刮拭，以痧痕出现为度。

2. 根据病情辨证刮拭配穴。涌泉穴可用隔衣刮痧法。

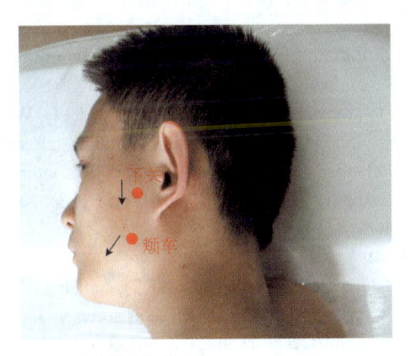

图128 下关、颊车
Fig.128 Xiaguan (ST 7) and Jiache (ST 6)

【注意事项】

1. 牙痛诊治前需明确诊断，注意及时治疗原发病。

2. 注意保持口腔卫生。

3. 调节生活起居，保证充足睡眠。少食刺激性食物及避免烟酒刺激。

Section 3 Toothache

Toothache is caused by one of the following factors: stagnant heat in the intestine and stomach, excessive ingestion of spicy or fried food, external contraction of wind-heat, up-rising of deficient fire due to yin deficiency (the aging process), unclean mouth cavity, and rotting teeth. It can be triggered by cold, heat, sweet, or sour stimulation.

[Major points] Jiache (ST 6), Xiaguan (ST 7), and Hegu (LI 4). (See Fig.59, 128)

[Point combination] For toothache due to wind-fire, combine Fengchi (GB 20), Waiguan (SJ 5), and Taiyang (EX-HN 5); for toothache due to stomach-fire, combine Quchi (LI 11), Waiguan (SJ 5), and Neiting (ST 44); for constipation, combine left-sided Guilai (ST 29) and left-sided Qichong (ST 30); and for toothache due to deficient fire, combine Sanyinjiao (SP 6), Taixi (KI 3), Xingjian (LR 2), and Yongquan (KI 1).

[Operation]

1. Press Jiache (ST 6), Xiaguan (ST 7), and Hegu (LI 4) with moderate or heavy force until the patient feels soreness and distension in the local area, and scrape Hegu (LI 4) towards the tip of index finger until Sha marks appear.

2. Scrape other points according to specific symptoms.
[Cautionary notes]
1. Be clear about the diagnosis and treat possible primary causes.
2. Keep the oral cavity clean.
3. Regulate the lifestyle, have adequate sleep, reduce food that causes irritation and stay away from cigarettes or alcohol.

第四节 咽喉肿痛

咽喉肿痛是口咽和喉咽肿胀、疼痛、吞咽不适为主要表现的临床病症。多由于感受风热外邪或过食辛辣煎炸食物或年老肾虚，阴亏火旺导致。

【主穴】廉泉、风府、风池、合谷。（图58、59、129）

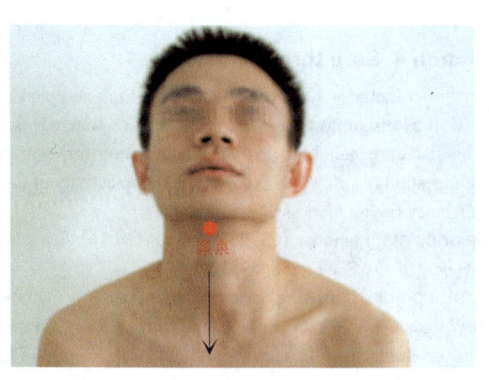

图129 廉泉
Fig.129 Lianquan (CV 23)

【配穴】外感风热配外关、鱼际、尺泽；胃火内炽配鱼际、内庭、行间；虚火上炎配三阴交、太溪、肾俞。

【操作方法】

1. 廉泉穴向胸骨上窝、颈根部刮拭，风府、风池穴向项后刮拭，以痧痕出现为度。

2. 合谷穴点揉至酸胀感，并向示指末端刮拭至痧痕出现。

3. 根据辨证刮拭配穴。

【注意事项】

1. 注意平日饮食起居调节。保持口腔卫生。避免烟酒辛辣煎炸刺激。

2. 对于重症患者，应及时进行综合治疗。

Section 4 Sore throat

Sore throat includes symptoms such as swelling and pain of the throat as well as discomfort on swallowing food or water. It is often caused by factors including external contraction of wind-heat, excessive ingestion of spicy or fried food, and hyperactivity of fire due to yin deficiency (aging process).

[Major points] Lianquan (CV 23), Fengfu (GV 16), Fengchi (GB 20), and Hegu (LI 4) .(See Fig.58, 59, 129)

[Point combination] For external contraction of wind-heat, combine Waiguan (SJ 5), Yuji (LU 10), and Chize (LU 5); for internal exuberance of stomach-fire, combine Yuji (LU 10), Neiting (ST 44), and Xingjian (LR 2); and for up-rising of deficient fire, combine Sanyinjiao (SP 6), Taixi (KI 3), and Shenshu (BL 23).

[Operation]

1. Scrape Lianquan (CV 23) towards the suprasternal fossa and collar area, and scrape Fengfu (GV 16) and Fengchi (GB 20) towards the nape until Sha marks appear.

2. Knead Hegu (LI 4) until the patient feels soreness and distension and then scrape towards the tip of index finger until the occurrence of Sha marks.

3. Scrape other points according to specific symptoms.

[Cautionary notes]

1. Regulate the dietary habits and lifestyle, keep the oral cavity clean, and stay away from cigarettes, alcohol, and spicy or fried food.

2. Those with a severe condition require comprehensive therapy.

第十三章　刮痧疗法在美容保健方面的应用

第一节　减肥

世界卫生组织（WHO）的标准，人体脂肪积聚过多，体重超过标准体重的10%为超重，20%以上为肥胖症。无明显的神经、内分泌或代谢病的单纯性肥胖在临床上最为多见。而继发性肥胖症则指继发于神经—内分泌—代谢紊乱，且与遗传或药物等有关。

【主穴】背俞穴、手三里、天枢、阴陵泉、丰隆。（图78、118、130～132）

【配穴】腹部肥胖者配中脘、滑肉门、左腹结；腰部肥胖者配章门、维道、肓门、胞肓、三焦俞；大腿肥胖者配髀关、伏兔、箕门、血海、风市；上臂肥胖者配肩贞、臂臑、天府；大便不畅或便秘配支沟、左腹结；肝郁气滞配期门、太冲；体虚或肝肾不足配三阴交、太溪、肾俞、气海。

【操作方法】

1. 背俞穴由上向下刮拭至骶部，以皮肤潮红为度。

2. 手三里刮向肘关节、天枢向腹下方、阴陵泉刮向胫骨内侧方向刮拭，至痧痕出现为止。

3. 根据病情辨证刮拭配穴，以皮肤泛红为度。

【注意事项】

1. 适当控制饮食，减少或忌食肥甘厚味，辛辣煎炸食物，忌零食。保持大便通畅。

2. 制定切合实际的体育锻炼或体力活动，并持之以恒。

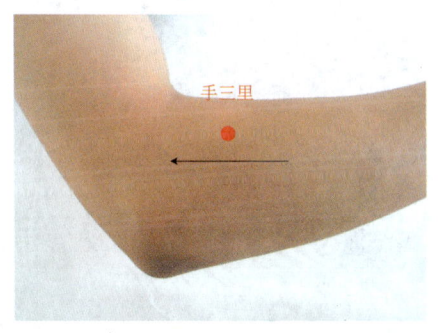

图130 手三里
Fig.130 Shousanli (LI 10)

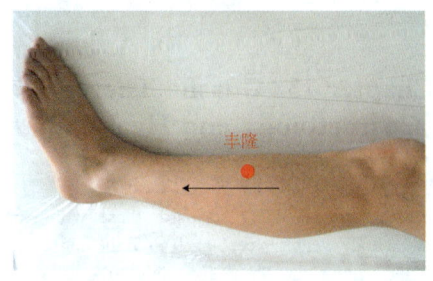

图131 丰隆
Fig.131 Fenglong (ST 40)

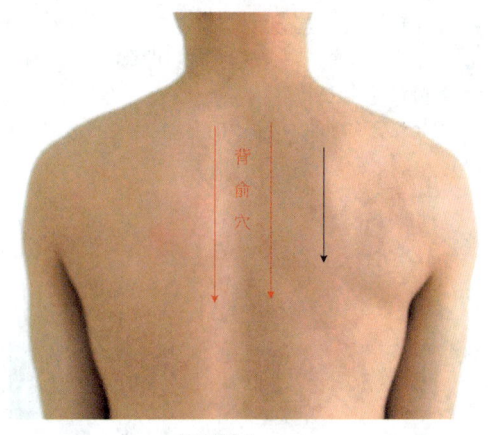

图132 背俞穴
Fig.132 back-Shu points

3. 注意肥胖症的诊断，对于继发性肥胖症应以治疗原发病症为先。

Chapter 13 Guasha Therapy for Cosmetology and Health Care

Section 1 Weight loss

According to the WHO standard, those with excessive fat deposits and a body weight exceeding 10% of the normal body weight are considered overweight. Those exceeding 20% of the normal body weight are considered as obesity. The simple obesity without significant nerve, endocrine, or metabolic diseases is more common. Secondary obesity is associated with nerve-endocrine-metabolism disorder, heredity or medication.

[Major points] Bach-Shu points, Shousanli (LI 10), Tianshu (ST 25), Yinlingquan (SP 9), and Fenglong (ST 40). (See Fig.78, 118, 130-132)

[Point combination] For abdominal fatness, combine Zhongwan (CV 12), Huaroumen (ST 24), and left-sided Fujie (SP 14); for waist enlargement, combine Zhangmen (LR 13), Weidao (GB 28), Huangmen (BL 51), Gaohuang (BL 53), and Sanjiaoshu (BL 22); for thigh fatness, combine Biguan (ST 31), Futu (ST 32), Jimen (SP 11), Xuehai (SP 10), and Fengshi (GB 31); for upper arm fatness, combine Jianzhen (SI 9), Binao (LI 14), and Tianfu (LU 3); for constipation, combine Zhigou (SJ 6) and left-sided Fujie (SP 14); for liver-qi stagnation, combine Qimen (LR 14) and Taichong (LR); and for weak constitution or deficiency of the liver and kidney, combine Sanyinjiao (SP 6), Taixi (KI 3), Shenshu (BL 23), and Qihai (CV 6).

[Operation]

1. Scrape back-Shu points downwards to the sacral region until the skin turns red.

2. Scrape Shousanli (LI 10) towards the elbow joint, scrape Tianshu (ST 25) towards the lower abdomen, and scrape Yinlingquan (SP 9) towards the medial aspect of the tibia until Sha marks appear.

3. Scrape other points according to specific symptoms until the skin turns red.

[Cautionary notes]

1. Limit food intake, reduce or avoid fatty, sweet, and fried food, stay away from snack food, and maintain smooth bowel movement.

2. Set a practical plan for physical exercise and persevere with it.

3. Be clear about the diagnosis and treat the primary cause for secondary obesity.

第二节 脱发

脱发是指毛发稀疏脱落或呈局限性脱落的一种常见病。脂溢性脱发多伴有皮脂溢出，脱发从前额向头顶发展，男性多见；斑秃，又称"鬼剃头"，常突然发生，迅速扩大，严重者累及身体其他部位毛发脱落。

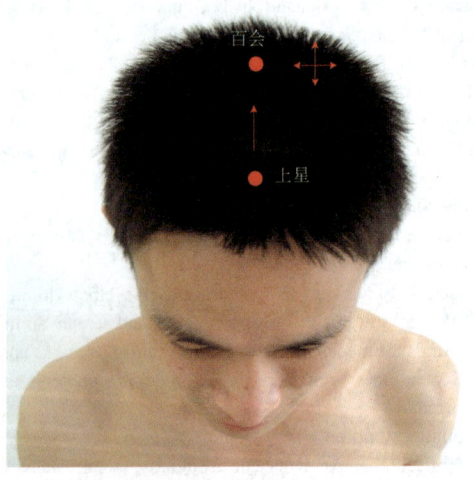

图133 百会、上星
Fig.133 Baihui (GV 20) and Shangxing (GV 23)

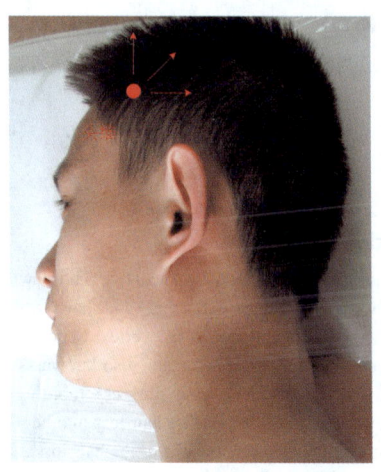

图134 头维
Fig.134 Touwei (ST 8)

【主穴】阿是穴（脱发部位）、头维、上星、风池、百会。（图58、133、134）

【配穴】体虚年老、肝肾不足者配肝俞、肾俞、三阴交、太溪，或背部脊柱两侧；外感风邪者配列缺、合谷、肺俞、膈俞。

【操作方法】

1. 先以中等力度刮拭阿是穴，至皮肤泛红。
2. 以轻、中力度从头维呈扇形、上星向头项后刮拭。
3. 以星状放射法刮拭百会穴，以局部热感为佳。
4. 根据病情刮拭配穴。

【注意事项】

1. 注意调节生活饮食起居情志。保持心情舒畅,定时休息,忌烟酒。

2. 对于某些药物或特殊治疗引起的脱发,刮痧疗法应在专业医生指导下,视具体情况而定。

Section 2 Hair loss

Hair loss can be general or localized. Those with seborrhoeic alopecia always experience seborrhea and hair loss starting from forehead and progressing towards the vertex. Seborrhoeic alopecia is more common in men. Alopecia areata, also known as 'a ghost hair cut', always occurs suddenly and progress rapidly. Those with a severe condition may also experience hair loss in other body parts.

[Major points] Ashi points (area of the hair loss), Touwei (ST 8), Shangxing (GV 23), Fengchi (GB 20), and Baihui (GV 20). (See Fig. 58, 133, 134)

[Point combination] For a weak constitution due to the aging process and deficiency of the liver and kidney, combine Ganshu (BL 18), Shenshu (BL 23), Sanyinjiao (SP 6), Taixi (KI 3), or bilateral sides of the spine; and for external contraction of wind, combine Lieque (LU 7), Hegu (LI 4), Feishu (BL 13), and Geshu (BL 17).

[Operation]

1. Scrape Ashi points with moderate force until the skin turns red.

2. Scrape Touwei (ST 8) with mild or moderate force in a fan shape and scrape Shangxing (GV 23) towards the nape.

3. Scrape Baihui (GV 20) in a star shape radiating away, until the patient has a warm sensation in the local area.

4. Scrape other points according to specific symptoms.

[Cautionary notes]

1. Regulate lifestyle and emotions, have adequate rest, and stay away from cigarettes or alcohol.

2. Consult a specialist for hair loss caused by medication or certain therapies.

第三节 痤疮

痤疮，又称为"青春痘"、"粉刺"，是指一种皮肤毛囊、皮脂腺的慢性炎症性病症。本病多由于外感风热、嗜食辛辣炙煿刺激之品，胃肠湿热蕴结或熬夜劳作、情绪波动、肝郁化火或妇女瘀热胞宫所致。

【主穴】大椎、肺俞、曲池、合谷、三阴交。（图57、76、135）

【配穴】外感风热者配外关；胃肠湿热者配阴陵泉、丰隆；肝胆火热者配太冲、阳陵泉；妇女瘀热胞宫者配太溪、次髎；大便不通者配左腹结、曲池、天枢。

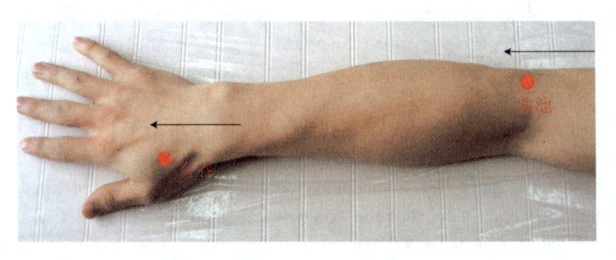

图135 合谷、曲池
Fig.135 Hegu (LI 4) and Quchi (LI 11)

【操作方法】

1. 先刮主穴至痧痕出现为度。

2. 根据临床病情辨证刮拭配穴。

【注意事项】

1. 注意饮食、起居、情志的调摄。多食蔬菜水果，保持大便通畅。

2. 注意保持面部皮肤清洁，禁止局部挤压。避免使用过于油腻或低劣、过期的化妆品。

Section 3　Acne

Acne, also known as 'pimples', refers to a chronic inflammatory condition of hair follicles and sebaceous glands of the skin. It is often caused by the following factors: external contraction of wind-heat, damp-heat accumulation in gastro-intestine due to excessive ingestion of spicy and fried food, liver-qi stagnation transforming into fire, or stagnant heat in the uterus.

[Major points] Dazhui (GV 14), Feishu (BL 13), Quchi (LI 11), Hegu (LI 4), and Sanyinjiao (SP 6) .(See Fig.57, 76, 135)

[Point combination] For external contraction of wind-heat, combine Waiguan (SJ 5); for damp-heat in the gastro-intestine, combine Yinlingquan (SP 9) and Fenglong (ST 40); for fire in the liver and gallbladder, combine Taichong (LR 3) and Yanglingquan (GB 34); for stagnant heat in the uterus, combine Taixi (KI 3) and Ciliao (BL 32); and for constipation, combine left-sided Fujie (SP 14), Quchi (LI 11), and Tianshu (ST 25).

[Operation]

1. Scrape major points first until Sha marks appear.
2. Scrape other points according to specific symptoms.
[Cautionary notes]
1. Regulate the diet, lifestyle and emotions, and eat more vegetables and fruits to keep smooth bowel movements.
2. Keep facial skin clean, avoid local squeezing, and stay away from oily, low-quality, or out of date cosmetic products.

第四节　保健养生刮痧法

人体的生长、发育、衰老与内在脏腑经络气血的功能状况有密切关系。刮痧疗法能刺激人体皮部络脉、体表腧穴，活血通络，平衡阴阳，提高机体的免疫功能，并通过经络的作用，起到良好的调整和防病保健作用。

【主穴】足三里、下巨虚、气海、关元、百会、四神聪、中脘、三阴交、太溪、涌泉。（图136～140）

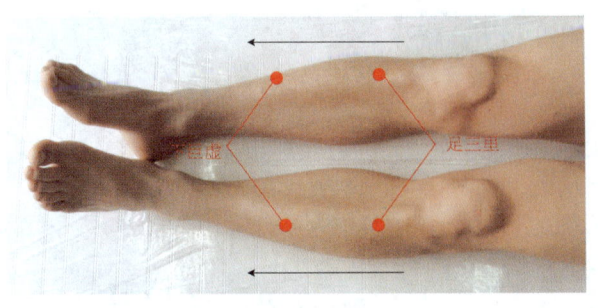

图136 足三里、下巨虚
Fig.136 Zusanli (ST 36) and Xiajuxu (ST 39)

下篇 刮痧疗法的实践应用
Part B Guasha Therapy in Practice

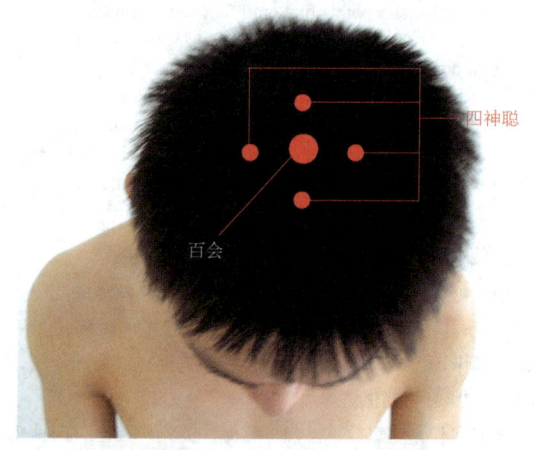

四神聪

百会

图137 百会、四神聪
Fig.137 Baihui (GV 20) and Sishencong (EX-HN 1)

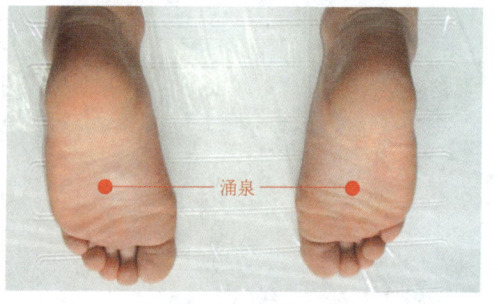

涌泉

图138 涌泉
Fig.138 Yongquan (KI 1)

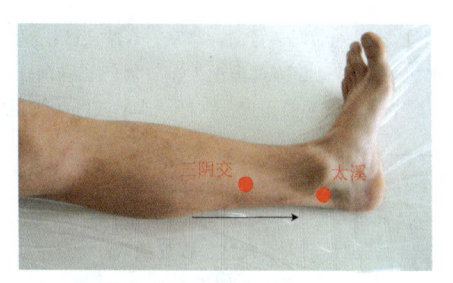

第十三章　刮痧疗法在美容保健方面的应用
Chapter 13　Guasha Therapy for Cosmetology and Health Care

图139 三阴交、太溪
Fig.139 Sanyinjiao (SP 6) and Taixi (KI 3)

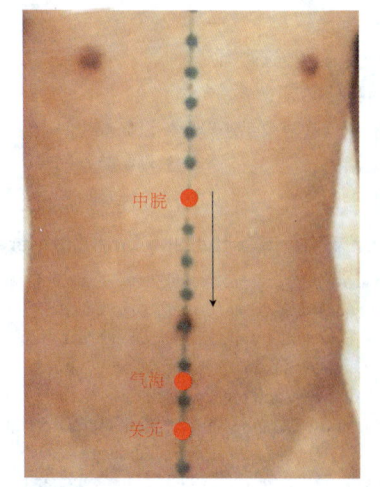

图140 中脘、气海、关元
Fig.140 Zhongwan (CV 12), Qihai (CV 6), and Guanyuan (CV 4)

【配穴】肾虚配命门、肾俞、志室、八髎穴区；脾虚配膈俞、胃俞、大包、章门；心肺气虚配大椎、风门、肺俞、膈俞、膻中；整体调节配大椎至腰阳关、大杼至八髎穴区，或相应的经脉循行线。

【操作方法】

1. 以轻缓、柔和的力度刮拭足三里至下巨虚、气海至关元、中脘至脐上、三阴交至太溪穴区，以皮肤微红为度。也可隔衣刮拭，直至局部微热而不损皮肤为宜。

2. 刮拭百会至四神聪可从百会向四神聪呈星状放射状刮拭，或隔布刮拭。

3. 根据自身体质选刮配穴。

【注意事项】

1. 保健刮痧法要求手法轻柔，以局部皮肤微红为度。

2. 可采用隔衣刮痧法，至局部皮肤微热即可。

Section 4 Guasha therapy for health preservation

Human growth, development, and aging are all closely related to qi and blood in zang-fu organs and meridians. Guasha therapy can stimulate the cutaneous collaterals and points and therefore activate blood, unblock collaterals, balance yin-yang, improve immune function, prevent potential diseases, and preserve health.

[Major points] Zusanli (ST 36), Xiajuxu (ST 39), Qihai (CV 6), Guanyuan (CV 4), Baihui (GV 20), Sishencong (EX-HN 1), Zhongwan (CV 12), Sanyinjiao (SP 6), Taixi (KI 3), and Yongquan (KI 1) .(See Fig. 136-140)

[Point combination] For kidney deficiency, combine Mingmen (GV 4), Shenshu (BL 23), Zhishi (BL 52), and Baliao area (bilateral BL 31-34); for spleen deficiency, combine Geshu (BL 17), Weishu (BL 21), Dabao (SP 21), and Zhangmen (LR 13); for qi deficiency of the heart and lung, combine Dazhui (GV 14), Fengmen (BL 12), Feishu (BL 13), Geshu (BL 17), and Danzhong (CV 17); and for general regulation, combine the area from Dazhui (GV 14) to Yaoyangguan (GV 3), from Dazhu (BL 11) to Baliao area (bilateral BL 31-34) or corresponding meridian pathway.

[Operation]

1. Scrape the area from Zusanli (ST 36) to Xiajuxu (ST 39), from Qihai (CV 6) to Guanyuan (CV 4), from Zhongwan (CV 12) to umbilicus, and from Sanyinjiao (SP 6) to Taixi (KI 3) with soft and moderate force until the skin turns slightly red; or scrape above areas with clothes on until a slight warm sensation occurs.

2. Scrape Baihui (GV 20) towards Sishencong (EX-HN 1) in a star or reflex shape or scrape with cloth-partition.

3. Scrape other points according to individual constitution.

[Cautionary notes]

1. Soft and gentle stimulation is advised for health-preservation and stop scraping should cease after the skin turns slightly red.

2. Guasha therapy over clothes can also be adopted until a slight warm sensation occurs in the local area.

附篇　刮痧疗法典型验案举隅
Attached chapter　Case Studies of Guasha Therapy

验案一　刮痧治疗失眠验案

李某，男，35岁，商人。3个月前于夜间睡眠时被电话吵醒，此后经常出现不易入睡，或睡眠时间短，或睡眠不深，甚者彻夜不眠的情况，就诊于神经内科，予安定镇静安眠，但用药1个月后睡眠未见明显改善且出现耐受性，故求诊我针灸科，因患者惧痛，故考虑予刮痧治疗，查体见：神志清楚，血压110/70mmHg，心肺腹未见异常，舌淡红苔薄黄，脉弦。

【主穴配穴】背部脊柱两旁、百会、印堂、神门、三阴交，配太冲、期门。

【操作方法】

1. 先刮拭脊柱两旁的背俞穴，重刮心俞、神堂、肝俞、魂门之间，以皮肤潮红即可。

2. 呈星状放射刮拭，从百会刮向四周，至局部温热感。

3. 印堂向上发根处刮拭、神门向上、三阴交向下刮拭至内踝后侧，以皮肤潮红为度。

4. 太冲向足趾末端，期门沿肋间向身体外侧刮拭，以皮肤潮红为度。

刮痧6次，配合中药调理，李某的睡眠质量明显改善，并坚持做保健刮痧，调理1个月后，患者告别失眠。

Case report 1 Guasha therapy for insomnia

Li, male, a 35-year-old businessman, complained of frequent difficulty falling asleep, a short sleep time, easily-disturbed sleep, or sometimes even sleeplessness throughout the night. This had occurred since he was woken by a telephone call during the night sleep 3 months ago. He was then treated with sleeping pills in the neurology department. However after 1 month of medication, he hadn't responded well to the sleeping pills and had developed a tolerance. Physical examination showed the following signs and symptoms: clear consciousness, blood pressure: 110/70mmHg, no abnormal signs of heart and lung conditions, a pale-red tongue with a thin, yellow coating, and a wiry pulse.

[Major points] Bilateral sides of the spine, Baihui (GV 20), Yintang (EX-HN 3), Shenmen (HT 7), Sanyinjiao (SP 6) [Point combination] Taichong (LR 3) and Qimen (LR 14).

[Operation]

1. Scrape the back-Shu points first, especially the area from Xinshu (BL 15), Shentang (BL 44), Ganshu (BL 18), and Hunmen (BL 47) until the skin turns red.

2. Scrape Baihui (GV 20) in four directions in a star shape until a warm sensation occurs in the local area.

3. Scrape Yintang (EX-HN 3) upwards to the hair root, Shenmen (HT 7) upwards, and Sanyinjiao (SP 6) downwards until the skin turns red.

4. Scrape Taichong (LR 3) towards the tips of the toes and scrape Qimen (LR 14) outwards along the intercostal space until the skin turns red.

[Result] After 6 Guasha treatments plus regulation of a Chinese herbal formula, the patient's sleep was significantly improved. After that he still continued the Guasha therapy for regulation. After another month, normal sleep was restored.

验案二 刮痧治疗胃痛验案

王某，女，28岁，教师。多年来因教学任务较重，故经常加班未能按时进食三餐，胃脘部时有隐痛，1个月前因上腹疼痛被诊断为上消化道溃疡，常规给予抑制胃酸分泌、保护胃黏膜药物治疗，但治疗期间仍时常发作，遂患者于发作期求诊我针灸科，查体：患者痛苦面容，双手捂上腹部痛处，血压100/68mmHg，心肺未见明显异常，上腹部压痛，无反跳痛，舌淡苔薄白，脉弦细。

【主穴配穴】梁丘、至阳、内关、足三里，配中脘、期门、脾俞、胃俞、肝俞。

【操作方法】

1. 梁丘、内关、足三里、中脘分别先点按至酸胀感，再刮拭至皮肤潮红或痧痕出现。

2. 期门沿肋间向身体外侧刮拭，以皮肤潮红为度。

3. 俯卧，刮拭脊柱两旁的背俞穴，重点刮拭脾俞、胃俞、肝俞以及至阳，至皮肤潮红为度。

刮痧10次，配合中药调理，王某的胃脘痛明显改善，并坚持做保健刮痧，调理3个月后，患者诉未再发。

Case report 2　Guasha therapy for gastric pain

Wang, female, a 28-year-old teacher, suffered from years of dull gastric pain due to irregular meals. She was diagnosed with an upper digestive tract ulcer last month because of upper abdominal pain. She was treated with medications that act to inhibit gastric acid secretion and protect the gastric mucosa. However she still experienced pain during the treatment course. Physical examination showed the following signs and symptoms: a dull complexion, a tendency to cover the upper abdomen with two hands, blood pressure: 100/68mmHg, no abnormal signs of heart and lung conditions, tenderness to palpation in the upper abdomen, no rebound tenderness, a pale tongue with a thin and white coating, and a wiry and thready pulse.

[Major points] Liangqiu (ST 34), Zhiyang (GV 9), Neiguan (PC 6), and Zusanli (ST 36). [Point combination] Zhongwan (CV 12), Qimen (LR 14), Pishu (BL 20), Weishu (BL 21), and Ganshu (BL 18).

[Operation]

1. Knead Liangqiu (ST 34), Neiguan (PC 6), Zusanli (ST 36), and Zhongwan (CV 12) until the patient feels soreness and distension and then scrape until the skin turns red or Sha marks appear.

2. Scrape Qimen (LR 14) outward along the intercostal space until the skin turns red.

3. Ask the patient to take prone position and scrape the back-Shu points, especially Pishu (BL 20), Weishu (BL 21), Ganshu (BL 18), and Zhiyang (GV 9) until the skin turns red.

[Result] After 10 Guasha treatments plus regulation with a Chinese herbal formula, the patient's gastric pain was significantly relieved. After that, the patient continued Guasha therapy for health preservation. After 3 months, the gastric pain completely ceased with no recurrence.

验案三 刮痧治疗落枕验案

廖某，男，26岁，IT职员。长期伏案工作，每天面对电脑工作的时间约9小时，近日来，为按期完成工作量加班熬夜，劳累困倦后伏于电脑桌上休息片刻，待清醒后发现颈项部强痛，酸胀难忍，且颈部活动受限，无明显的手臂部麻木等异常感觉，求诊我针灸门诊，查体：颈项部肌肉紧张，无法完成颈椎生理范围内的活动。臂丛神经牵拉试验阴性，舌淡苔薄白，脉弦。

【主穴配穴】患侧风池、肩井、风门、天宗、落枕穴。配外关、后溪。

【操作方法】

1. 先刮患侧风池至肩井穴区，再刮风池、风门穴，至出现痧痕为止。

2. 天宗、落枕穴先点揉至酸胀感，再刮拭，以痧痕出现为度。

3. 沿前臂长轴向上肢远端呈线状刮拭外关穴，并用点状刮拭后溪穴，直到出现痧痕为度。

刮痧3次，廖某的颈项部疼痛活动受限的症状消除，嘱其注意休息、局部保暖。

Case report 3 Guasha therapy for stiff neck

Liao, male, a 26-year-old IT clerk, who works with a computer for approximately 9 hours every day, complained of intolerable neck soreness, stiffness, and pain, along with limited neck movement after sleeping at the computer desk due to overwork in recent days. He had no significant numbness of hands and arms. Physical examination showed tense cervical muscles and an inability to fulfill physiological motor range of cervical vertebra. The brachial plexus nerve pulling test was negative. His tongue is pale with thin and white coating and his pulse is wiry.

[Major points] Fengchi (GB 20), Jianjing (GB 21), Fengmen (BL 12), Tianzong (SI 11), and Luozhen (Extra) in the affected side.
[Point combination] Waiguan (SJ 5) and Houxi (SI 3)

[Operation]

1. Scrape the area from Fengchi (GB 20) to Jianjing (GB 21) on the affected side, and then scrape Fengchi (GB 20) and Fengmen (BL 12) until the skin turns red.

2. Knead Tianzong (SI 11) and Luozhen (Extra) until the patient feels soreness and distension and then scrape until the Sha marks appear.

3. Scrape Waiguan (SJ 5) in a linear shape along the long axis of the forearm and scrape Houxi (SI 3) in punctiform until Sha marks appear.

[Result] After 3 Guasha treatments, the patient's neck pain and limitation of neck movement disappeared. He was advised to take rest and keep the neck area warm.

验案四 刮痧治疗便秘验案

吴某，男，60岁。近半年来，大便涩滞，秘结不通，经常5~6天才排便一次，且每次排便的时间长达约1小时，每次排便都大汗淋漓，便质较硬，色常，量适中，小便正常，饮食正常，舌淡苔薄白，脉沉细。

【主穴配穴】天枢、左腹结、大肠俞、上巨虚、支沟，配脾俞、命门、肾俞、太溪。

【操作方法】

1. 左腹结向腹股沟方向，天枢穴、上巨虚向下，支沟穴向腕部方向刮拭，太溪穴点状刮拭，以皮肤潮红或至痧痕出现为止。

2. 脾俞、命门、肾俞、大肠俞向骶部刮拭、直至皮肤潮红或痧痕出现。

刮痧治疗8次，嘱患者进食药膳，平素多食水果蔬菜等富含水分和纤维的食物，并养成按时登厕排便的习惯，排便前后自行进行脐周按摩，以局部热感为度。经调理治疗后，患者可每3天排便一次，登厕时间也明显缩短。

Case report 4 Guasha therapy for constipation

Wu, male, 60 years old, complained of constipation for the last six months, one bowel movement every 5-6 days, each bowel movement lasting more than 1 hour with profuse sweating, hard stools with normal color and volume. The patient had normal urine and appetite. His tongue was pale with a thin and white coating and his pulse was wiry and deep.

[Major points] Tianshu (ST 25), left-sided Fujie (SP 14), Dachangshu (BL 25), Shangjuxu (ST 37), and Zhigou (SJ 6). [Point combination] Pishu (BL 20), Mingmen (GV 4), Shenshu (BL 23), and Taixi (KI 3).

[Operation]

1. Scrape left-sided Fujie (BL 20) towards the groin, scrape Tianshu (ST 25) and Shangjuxu (ST 37) downwards, scrape Zhigou (SJ 6) towards the wrist, and scrape Taixi (KI 3) in punctiform until the skin turns red.

2. Scrape Pishu (BL 20), Mingmen (GV 4), Shenshu (BL 23),

and Dachangshu (BL 25) towards the sacral region until the skin turns red or Sha marks appear.

[Result] The patient was treated with 8 Guasha treatments. In addition, he was advised to eat more fruits and vegetables that are rich in water and fiber, and go to the bathroom at regular times. He was also asked to massage the abdominal area around umbilicus until local area becomes warm before and after the bowel movement. After the treatment and regulation, the patient had one bowel movement every 3 days, and the time taken for each bowel movement was significantly shortened.

验案五 刮痧治疗月经不调验案

邓某，女，30岁。近3年来，月经周期紊乱，反复出现月经提早或推迟1周左右，经量适中、色暗红、质稠、伴较多血块，经期前几天多出现下腹部胀满、心烦易怒、夜寐不安，舌淡苔薄黄，脉弦涩。

【主穴配穴】合谷、膈俞、关元、归来、三阴交，配太冲、八髎穴区。

【操作方法】

1. 关元、归来刮向阴部毛际前，以皮肤潮红为度。

2. 合谷、三阴交、太冲先点按，再刮拭至皮肤潮红。

3. 八髎区向尾骶部。

每周刮痧治疗2次，持续治疗4个月，并嘱其注意经期的饮食、情绪调摄，治疗后患者自觉经色、经质都有明显的改善，睡眠、情绪等症状均有明显的好转。

Case report 5 Guasha therapy for irregular menstruation

Deng, female, 30 years old, had an irregular menstrual cycle for the last 3 years with recurrent early or delayed period (about one week), moderate menstrual volume, dark-red in color and thick in property, along with blood clots. Other symptoms and signs include lower abdominal fullness and distension, restlessness, irritability, poor sleep, a pale tongue with a thin and yellow coating, and a wiry and hesitant pulse.

[Major points] Hegu (LI 4), Geshu (BL 17), Guanyuan (CV 4), Guilai (ST 29), and Sanyinjiao (SP 6). [Point combination] Taichong (LR 3) and Baliao (bilateral BL 31-34).

[Operation]

1. Scrape Guanyuan (CV 4) and Guilai (ST 29) downwards to the pubic hairy region until the skin turns red.

2. Knead Hegu (LI 4), Sanyinjiao (SP 6), and Taichong (LR 3) first and then scrape until the skin turns red.

3. Scrape Baliao (bilateral BL 31-43) towards the caudal-sacral region.

[Result] The patient was treated with Guasha therapy for 4 months, twice each week. In addition, the patient was also advised to regulate the diet and emotion during menstruation. After the 4-month treatment course, the patient felt significant improvement in menstrual color and quality. Her sleep and emotions were also significantly improved.

验案六 刮痧治疗小儿消化不良验案

陶某,男,6岁。偏嗜零食,常于餐间进食大量不易消化的食物,每临三餐便不吃饭,一周以来,自觉脘腹部胀满疼痛,嗳气,时有呕吐,大便溏薄,舌淡苔厚腻,脉弦滑。

【主穴配穴】梁门、天枢、足三里、四缝,配内关、脾俞、胃俞。

【操作方法】

1. 先刮梁门至大枢、足三里向踝关节方向刮拭,以皮肤泛红为度;四缝,取2～3处,以痧发至痧痕出现为度。

2. 合谷、内关可用点揉法,再沿脊椎两旁从上向下刮,重刮脾俞、胃俞穴,以皮肤潮红为度。

刮痧治疗6次,结合控制餐间滥食零食,饮食定时定量,避免生冷、油腻等,患者于治疗后可进食正常食量饮食,无脘腹部胀满感,无呕吐,便质如常。

Case report 6 Guasha therapy for infantile dyspepsia

Tao, a six-year old boy, loves snack food and frequently eats large amounts of difficult-to-digest food in between meals and hardly eats anything at meal times. He complained of gastric distension, fullness, and pain for one week, along with belching, occasional vomiting, loose stools, a pale tongue with a thick, greasy coating, and a wiry, slippery pulse.

[Major points] Liangmen (ST 21), Tianshu (ST 25), Zusanli (ST 36), Sifeng (EX-UE 10). [Point combination] Neiguan (PC 6),

Pishu (BL 20), and Weishu (BL 21).

[Operation]

1. Scrape Liangmen (ST 21) to Tianshu (ST 25) and Zusanli (ST 36) towards the ankle joint until the skin turns red; and select 2-3 points of Sifeng (EX-UE 10) until Sha marks appear.

2. Knead Hegu (LI 4) and Neiguan (PC 6), and then scrape the bilateral sides of the spine in a downwards direction, especially on Pishu (BL 20) and Weishu (BL 21) with heavy force until the skin turns red.

[Result] After 6 Guasha treatments plus limitation of snack food as well as raw, cold, and oily food, the boy began to normally with normal stools. The symptoms such as gastric fullness and distension and vomiting ceased.

参考文献

[1] 李琳,穆腊梅.中国民间疗法丛书－刮痧疗法[M].北京:中国中医药出版社，1994

[2] 王敬,杨金生.中国刮痧健康法378种病症临床治疗大全[M].北京:中国医药科技出版社，1994

[3] 潘金友.经穴刮痧疗百病[M].上海:上海中医药大学出版社，1998

[4] 金春乐,金春城,金春瑢.中国民间医学丛书－中国民间刮痧术[M].成都:四川科学技术出版社，1993

[5] 石学敏.针灸推拿学[M].北京:中国中医药出版社，1996

[6] 曲立彦,李淑云,陈华琴.图解刮痧疗法[M].北京:中国中医药出版社，1998

[7] 程爵棠,程功文.刮痧疗法治百病[M].北京:人民军医出版社，1999

Reference

1. Li Lin, Mu La-mei, Collections of China Folk Therapeutics on Guasha [M], Beijing: China Publishing House of Traditional Chinese Medicine, 1994
2. Wang Jing, Yang Jin-sheng, China Guasha Healthcare Methods on 378 Condition in Clinical Practice [M], Beijing: China Medical Science & Technology Press, 1994
3. Pan Jin-you, Treatment of A Hundred Diseases with Meridian Guasha Therapy [M], Shanghai: Press of Shanghai University of Traditional Chinese Medicine, 1998
4. Jin Chun-le, Jin Chun-e, Jin Chun-rong, Collections of China Folk Therapeutics on Folk Gua Therapy [M], Chengdu: Sichuan Publishing House of Science & Technology, 1993
5. Shi Xue-min, Science of Acupuncture and Tuina [M], Beijing: China Publishing House of Traditional Chinese Medicine, 1996
6. Qu Li-yan, Li Shu-yun, Chen Hua-qin, Guasha Therapy with Illustrations [M], Beijing: China Publishing House of Traditional Chinese Medicine, 1998
7. Cheng Jue-tang, Cheng Gong-wen, Miraculous Guasha Therapy [M], Beijing: People's Military Medical Press, 1999